101 Tips

for
Raising
Healthy Kids
with
Diabetes

Laura Hieronymus, MSEd, APRN, BC-ADM, CDE
Patti Geil, MS, RD, FADA, CDE

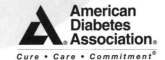

**American
Diabetes
Association.**

Cure • Care • Commitment®

Director, Book Publishing, John Fedor; *Managing Editor, Book Publishing,* Abe Ogden; *Associate Director, Consumer Books,* Robert Anthony; *Production Manager,* Melissa Sprott; *Cover Design,* Koncept, Inc.; *Printer,* Worzalla Publishing.

Printed in the United States of America
1 3 5 7 9 10 8 6 4 2

The suggestions and information contained in this publication are generally consistent with the *Clinical Practice Recommendations* and other policies of the American Diabetes Association, but they do not represent the policy or position of the Association or any of its boards or committees. Reasonable steps have been taken to ensure the accuracy of the information presented. However, the American Diabetes Association cannot ensure the safety or efficacy of any product or service described in this publication. Individuals are advised to consult a physician or other appropriate health care professional before undertaking any diet or exercise program or taking any medication referred to in this publication. Professionals must use and apply their own professional judgment, experience, and training and should not rely solely on the information contained in this publication before prescribing any diet, exercise, or medication. The American Diabetes Association—its officers, directors, employees, volunteers, and members—assumes no responsibility or liability for personal or other injury, loss, or damage that may result from the suggestions or information in this publication.

The paper in this publication meets the requirements of the ANSI Standard Z39.48-1992 (permanence of paper).

∞ ADA titles may be purchased for business or promotional use or for special sales. To purchase this book in large quantities, or for custom editions of this book with your logo, contact Lee Romano Sequeira, Special Sales & Promotions, at the address below, or at LRomano@diabetes.org or 703-299-2046.

American Diabetes Association
1701 North Beauregard Street
Alexandria, Virginia 22311

Library of Congress Cataloging-in-Publication Data
Hieronymus, Laura.
    101 tips for raising healthy kids with diabetes / Laura Hieronymus, Patti Geil.
        p. cm.
    Includes bibliographical references and index.
    ISBN 1-58040-242-9 (alk. paper)
    1. Diabetes in children–Popular works. 2. Diabetes in children–Patients–Care. I. Title: One hundred one tips for raising healthy kids with diabetes. II. Geil, Patti Bazel. III. Title.

    RJ420.D5H44 2006
    618.92'462–dc22
                                        2006003188

To my daughters, Kelly and Lindsay—you are the root of mine and Dad's heart.

To my parents, Tommy and Marguerite Bertram, for raising this healthy kid, not only with diabetes, but with love.

To Tom Brodie and Larry Smith, two dads who are champions for the cause of diabetes.

-Laura

101 heartfelt thanks to my parents, Ed and Irene Bazel, who taught me everything I know about raising healthy kids.

101 hugs and kisses to my husband Jack and daughters Kristen and Rachel, who continue to teach me about raising healthy kids every day!

-Patti

...and to all kids with diabetes in the Central Kentucky Bluegrass area, as well as their parents. We appreciate the teaching and learning we share as a team.

-Patti & Laura

CONTENTS

Preface vii

CHAPTER

1   Off to a Healthy Start! 1

2   Bouncing Babies to Terrific Toddlers 13

3   Preschool to Primary School:
ABC's of Management 21

4   School-Aged Children:
Adding Confidence, Subtracting Fear 29

5   Adolescents:
Maturity Matters with Metabolism. 35

6   Healthy Eating for Healthy Kids. 43

7   The Art and Science of Medication
Management 55

8   Child's Play:
Physical Activity and Exercise 65

9   Monitoring:
Checking Up on Blood Glucose Control 73

10   Psychosocial:
Living and Coping with Diabetes 85

11   School Days:
Factoring Diabetes into the Equation. 93

12   Athletes with Diabetes:
Champions and Challenges 101

13   Special Events:
No Kid-ding Around 107

14   Ongoing Care:
Successful Diabetes Self-Management. 115

Index 125

PREFACE

A child is the root of the heart.
–Maria de Jesus

There is no greater love than that of a parent for his or her child. So when the challenge of a chronic illness, such as diabetes, enters a child's life, it becomes a challenge for the parent, as well. In fact, when a child has diabetes, it affects all of those around him or her, from grandparents to school teachers to best friends. Whether newly diagnosed or having lived with diabetes for several years, ongoing learning and new information is essential because as kids grow, diabetes care needs change. Despite the advances in diabetes care in the last decade, dealing with diabetes still requires a great deal of attention and skill in its day-to-day management.

Diabetes is the most common chronic illness in youth. In the population under 20 years of age, it is estimated that 176,500, or 0.22%, have diabetes. About one in every 400–600 children and adolescents has type 1 diabetes. Type 2 diabetes, until recently, was thought to be primarily a disease in adults. However, today, cases of type 2 diabetes are being diagnosed more and more frequently in youth, particularly American Indians, African Americans, and Hispanic/Latino Americans.

101 Tips for Raising Healthy Kids with Diabetes is inspired by commonly asked questions from those parents whose children, ranging from infants to adolescents, are dealing with the diagnosis and management of diabetes. As diabetes educators with years of professional experience in diabetes self-management education as well as expertise in the ups and downs of diabetes care in youth, we welcome the opportunity to share with you our answers to these questions. It is our hope that all kids grow up to become happy, healthy adults, including those who just happen to have diabetes.

Chapter 1.
Off to a Healthy Start!

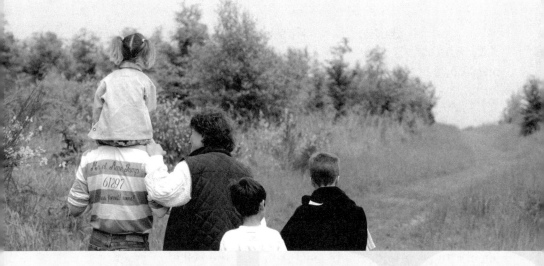

*T*he diagnosis of diabetes in a child brings changes and challenges to the lives of everyone involved. Rest assured that you will master the seemingly overwhelming amount of important information you are facing. With a healthy start, you will soon find the individualized approach to diabetes care that works best for your child and your entire family.

One

My child has always had a "sweet tooth." Did this cause his diabetes?

Eating sugar and sweets does not cause diabetes. This is a common myth that's simply not true. Research is still being done, but no one knows exactly why children develop diabetes. Type 1 diabetes, formerly known as juvenile-onset diabetes, is the result of the body's autoimmune system attacking the insulin-producing cells in the pancreas. Insulin is a hormone that helps cells in the body convert glucose into energy. Without insulin, the glucose remains in the blood and rises to dangerous levels. Type 2 diabetes used to be known as adult-onset diabetes, but is being diagnosed more and more often in children. In type 2 diabetes, the body either does not produce enough insulin or the cells ignore it (a condition known as insulin resistance), with the result being the same as type 1 diabetes—glucose is unable to move from the bloodstream into the cells for energy.

Many researchers believe diabetes is the result of both genetics and environmental factors. Genes and family history play a big part in the development of diabetes, particularly with type 2 diabetes. However, genetics is not the only factor. The majority of children who develop type 1 diabetes have no family history of the condition, which seems to suggest there might be some sort of outside trigger that causes the body to destroy its own insulin-making cells. Environment can also affect the development of type 2 diabetes, which is associated with obesity, lack of physical activity, or a family history of diabetes.

Two

The pediatrician says my 12-year-old daughter has "adult-onset diabetes," but she's just a child. How can that be?

Your daughter has type 2 diabetes, which used to be known as adult-onset diabetes, though this is no longer the case because type 2 is being more commonly diagnosed in young people. It's felt that this dramatic increase in diagnosis is related to the rise in the incidence of obesity in young people, which has increased by almost 50% over the past 20 years.

In type 2 diabetes, either the body does not produce enough insulin or the cells ignore it, with the result being that glucose is unable to move from the bloodstream into the cells for energy. These high blood glucose levels have immediate consequences, such as fatigue, excessive thirst, hunger, urination, and blurry vision. High blood glucose also has potential long-term consequences, such as damage to the eyes, kidneys, nerves, and heart.

Treatment of type 2 in children is usually based on lifestyle changes, such as increased physical activity and healthy eating. Medication may be used if necessary. Losing weight will help keep blood glucose levels as close as possible to the target range. Treatment for type 2 diabetes in young people is most successful when the entire family is involved in making permanent lifestyle changes.

Three

Is there a cure for diabetes?

There is no "cure" for diabetes, although advances in treatment have made managing the disease more effective and made it possible for children with diabetes to live longer, healthier, and happier lives.

There are a number of possible cures being researched. Pancreas transplants are being explored as one avenue to cure type 1 diabetes. A healthy pancreas or even an artificial pancreas should enable the body to produce insulin again. However, the current medication regimen required to keep the body from rejecting the pancreas is nearly as arduous as treating diabetes. Also, there aren't nearly enough donors to make this a true option at this time.

Children with type 2 diabetes can manage their condition with medication and lifestyle changes, such as healthy eating and physical activity, but this isn't considered a true cure that makes the disease disappear.

A cure may not be available right now, but we do know that controlling blood glucose is the best way to prevent problems down the road. Results from studies such as the Diabetes Control and Complications Trial (DCCT) have proven that keeping blood glucose levels in good control lowers the incidence of diabetes complications. Until a cure can be found, the best approach is to keep blood glucose levels near target range by helping your child follow a diabetes treatment plan that includes healthy eating, physical activity, blood glucose monitoring, and medication if necessary.

Four

My aunt had diabetes and always had problems with her vision, kidneys, and circulation. What can I do to prevent this from happening to my son?

Try to keep blood glucose levels as close to normal as possible. Complications such as eye, kidney, nerve, or heart disease rarely appear in children, but it is important for your son to keep his glucose levels in good control today to lower the risk of these complications in the future. Research from an important study—the Diabetes Control and Complications Trial (DCCT)—proves that keeping blood glucose levels within target range with intensive treatment lowers the risk of eye disease by as much as 76%, kidney disease by 35-56%, and nerve damage by 60%. Although this study didn't include children younger than age 13, it makes sense that these results could apply.

Intensive treatment is defined as basal/bolus insulin therapy, using multiple daily insulin injections, or use of an insulin pump, checking blood glucose at least four times daily, and frequent visits with the diabetes care team. Intensive treatment does carry risks, including excess weight gain and hypoglycemia. Hypoglycemia is of special concern in younger children since it not only affects brain function immediately, it can also interfere with normal brain development if it is severe and frequent. Also remember that perfect blood glucose levels at every moment of the day are difficult to achieve and maintain without paying a high cost of energy, money, and stress, particularly in young children.

Five

Our teenage daughter is a sports fanatic. She was just diagnosed with type 1 diabetes. Can she still participate in soccer and basketball?

Yes, she can. Athletes with diabetes are active at all levels of organized sports, from recreational to professional. Your daughter can safely play any organized sport if you keep a few factors in mind:

- Your doctor will probably need to lower her insulin for periods when she is more active. Work with your diabetes care team on how much she should adjust her insulin for activity.
- All physical activity lowers blood glucose as it moves glucose from the bloodstream into working muscles. Various factors, including the intensity and duration of the activity, will influence the way in which a specific sport affects diabetes.
- Be prepared for the risk of hypoglycemia. Your daughter should check her blood glucose before practice and games and eat a small snack if necessary. Also, it's important to check blood glucose throughout the game or practice and immediately if symptoms of low blood glucose occur.
- Encourage your daughter to wear some form of medical alert identification that indicates she has diabetes. Her coaches and perhaps a teammate or two also need to know that she has diabetes and a few basic facts about blood glucose checks, symptoms and treatment of hypoglycemia, and the need for extra food.

Six

We know it's important to give insulin injections and check our 3-year-old son's blood glucose frequently. What can we do to make these "sticks" less traumatic?

There are a variety of ways. Preschoolers still can't completely understand why they must have injections and finger sticks. Naturally, they may be frightened by these "sticks" and may even see them as a punishment.

The best approach is a positive one. Acknowledge your son's fears by saying "Yes, I know it hurts," and, "You're being very brave." Rather than telling him he needs his shot because he is "sick," try the positive message that daily injections and finger sticks help him stay healthy.

Give your son a much-needed feeling of control over the situation to help ease his anxiety. Let him choose which finger to use for his finger stick or pick the spot for his insulin injection. Have him help you complete the procedure in whatever way he can.

Stickers and rewards encourage a child to have a finger stick or shot. You might set up a chart where your son earns a star for each finger stick or shot. The stars can be "redeemed" for a trip to the playground, an extra bedtime story, or another favorite treat.

Play therapy can also help your son deal with the anxiety. It may help if he pretends his favorite stuffed animal has diabetes and needs an insulin injection, too!

Try to maintain a positive outlook and keep in mind that the trauma of injections and finger sticks will diminish over time.

Seven

Our 8 year old is a picky eater. Now that she's been diagnosed with diabetes, how can we be sure she'll get enough to eat?

The simple answer is to let her appetite, growth, and blood glucose control be your guide.

- Adopt a positive attitude at meal and snack time. Be a good role model and eat the foods you'd like to see her eat. The job of the parent is to put the proper food choices on the table and your daughter's job is to be responsible for what and how much she eats.

- Have some backup choices for those times when pickiness sets in. You can offer easy-to-fix items such as grilled cheese sandwiches or peanut butter and crackers quickly if your child doesn't want to eat what you've prepared.

- Involve your daughter in menu planning, food shopping, and preparing fun recipes. If the meal is something she's planned or prepared, she'll be more likely to enjoy it. Check out *Cooking Up Fun for Kids with Diabetes*, published by the American Diabetes Association (ADA).

- If you are concerned about hypoglycemia, you may want to give your daughter her mealtime insulin after she eats, rather than before. This allows you to base her insulin dose on the amount she actually ate, lowering her risk for low blood glucose. Check with your diabetes care team for guidance.

- Don't forget to accentuate the positive by praising your daughter for eating well.

Eight

My pediatrician wants our family to see a diabetes educator. Is this important?

Yes. With a chronic condition such as diabetes you need to know as much as you can, because although the medical team develops your child's diabetes treatment plan, you and your family are responsible for nearly all of the daily care. A diabetes educator can teach you everything from basic survival skills to detailed ongoing education.

A certified diabetes educator (CDE) has met highly specialized academic, professional, and experience requirements and can be your coach and teacher throughout the process of making changes in your child and family's behavior and lifestyle. A diabetes educator may be a registered nurse, registered dietitian, pharmacist, physician, mental health professional, podiatrist, or exercise physiologist.

You and your family will become the true experts on your child's diabetes over time, but working with a diabetes educator can help you keep your knowledge up-to-date and accurate. You can find a diabetes educator near you by accessing the website of the American Association of Diabetes Educators, *www.diabeteseducator.org*. The American Diabetes Association also recognizes programs that meet the National Standards for excellence in diabetes education. You can find a program near you by accessing the website of the American Diabetes Association at *www.diabetes.org*.

Nine

As a parent of a child with diabetes, I often find myself feeling overwhelmed and frightened about my responsibility for her care. Is this normal?

A bsolutely. It is the rare parent that doesn't feel overwhelmed at times! Know that these feelings are normal and try not to maintain a negative outlook. A few tips for dealing with your feelings:

- Acquire knowledge. As you learn more about diabetes, you'll find yourself more confident in your abilities to manage the condition. Involve your child as much as possible so you are working together to gain control and beat diabetes.
- Anger that diabetes has entered your life is another normal reaction. Your child is probably angry, too. Talk about your feelings together and choose to accept them and move on.
- Guilt is a common emotion in parents of children with diabetes. Know that there's nothing you or your child have done to cause the condition or could have done to prevent it.
- Find a support group of parents and children who have "been there" and are living successfully with diabetes. Contact your local ADA office to find a support group in your area.
- Don't hesitate to get professional help for depression. Warning signs include apathy, trouble sleeping, eating problems, poor concentration, frequent crying, fatigue, anxiety, and even considering dying or hurting yourself. A counselor can work with you and your family to improve your outlook and ability to successfully live with diabetes.

Ten

Did my child inherit diabetes from me? Are our other children at risk?

Maybe. Diabetes does appear to be passed on through the genes, but research to date shows that it doesn't seem to be inherited in a straightforward fashion and the type of diabetes makes a difference. In both types, an individual must inherit a predisposition to diabetes and then something in the environment must trigger the development of the disease.

In type 1 diabetes, the immune system attacks the insulin-producing cells of the pancreas. While genetic factors may predispose someone to type 1 diabetes, an outside factor is required to trigger the disease. In other words, someone may have the gene for type 1 diabetes but never be exposed to the environmental trigger and thus never develop the disease.

Type 2 diabetes is more strongly associated with genetics. Children who have a parent with type 2 diabetes are much more likely to develop the disease. However, other things influence the development of type 2, particularly obesity, inactivity, and ethnic background. Type 2 diabetes is also more likely to occur in African Americans, Hispanics, Native Americans, and Pacific Islanders. Improving lifestyle choices lowers the risk of developing type 2 diabetes. If your child has type 2 diabetes, his siblings are at increased risk for the condition as well. Have the entire family follow the same recommendations for healthy eating and increased physical activity.

Chapter 2.
Bouncing Babies to Terrific Toddlers

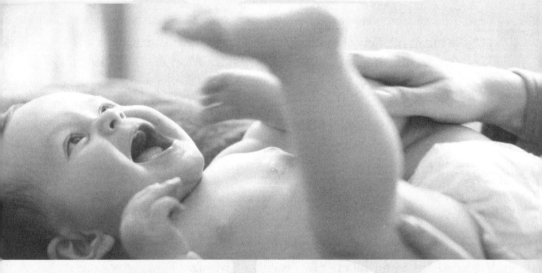

*B*abies with diabetes grow up to become terrific toddlers with the help of a loving family and a dedicated diabetes care team. However, infants and toddlers present their caregivers with a variety of challenges along the way. Just like children who don't have diabetes, infants and toddlers with diabetes are developing a trusting relationship with their caregivers, learning to communicate effectively, and striving for independence.

Eleven

How can I tell if my baby is having low blood glucose or is just feeling irritable?

Unfortunately, there is no clear-cut way to tell if your baby is suffering from hypoglycemia or just irritable. *When in doubt, treat for hypoglycemia.* The warning signs for hypoglycemia include:

- Crying or a particular cry that is different from that for a wet diaper or general crankiness
- Pale skin
- Bluish tinge to fingers or lips
- Irritability
- Sweating
- Trembling

Hypoglycemia in an infant is especially worrisome since babies aren't able to verbally tell their parents how they feel. Severe hypoglycemia can be potentially dangerous both short term (seizures and coma) and long term, since frequent hypoglycemia can affect brain development. Because of this, your diabetes care team may set target blood glucose levels for your baby a bit higher than those for older children.

Check your baby's blood glucose immediately if you suspect hypoglycemia and treat it with easily absorbed carbohydrate. If you can't do a blood glucose check, treat him anyway to ensure that his blood glucose doesn't stay low for too long. In this case, it's better to err on the side of running higher blood glucose levels for a short time.

Twelve

Should I wake my sleeping baby up to check her blood glucose level?

This depends on the day the baby has had. No one likes to wake a sleeping baby and in most cases you won't need to do a blood glucose check during naptime. However, if your baby has had an especially active day (learning to crawl, for example), you should pay extra attention to the amount you feed her as well as any symptoms of hypoglycemia. A baby monitor can also alert you to the sounds of a restless sleeper, another indication of hypoglycemia.

Because babies can't take in large quantities of food at one time, infants with diabetes often need middle-of-the-night feedings until they are able to take in enough calories and carbohydrate to last through the night. If your baby wakes for a feeding, you may want to take the opportunity to check her glucose. Avoid doing checks and injections in the baby's crib so she can always feel that her crib is a "safe" place.

While not as accurate as blood glucose testing, one alternative is to test a wet diaper for urine glucose by pulling some of the wet lining out of the diaper, pushing it into an empty syringe, and using the syringe plunger to squeeze out a drop of urine. A few cotton balls in the diaper can also be used to collect urine drops. These drops can be placed on a urine test strip and read.

Thirteen

What's the best way to treat low blood glucose in a baby?

Many of the hypoglycemia treatments that work for children work for babies and toddlers as well. Suggestions for treatment include:

- Easily absorbed liquid such as apple juice, sugar water, or another favorite beverage
- Glucose gel, syrup, or regular jelly placed on a soft toothbrush and rubbed into the gums
- Glucagon injections, which can be used when blood glucose is dangerously low and immediate action is needed (have your diabetes care team instruct you on using glucagon before an emergency occurs so you are well prepared in advance)

Babies with diabetes probably won't require as much carbohydrate as an older child to raise blood glucose; one ounce of juice or a teaspoon of syrup may do the trick. Fifteen minutes after treating for hypoglycemia, check your baby's blood glucose again to see if it has risen into the safe target range determined by your diabetes care team. Follow up with formula or solid food.

Fourteen

Is there a special type of insulin we need to use for our 9-month-old daughter?

There are no insulins specifically designed for babies. However, managing insulin regimens in infants is especially challenging. Their unpredictable appetites and the fact that they eat and drink small amounts frequently throughout the day leads many doctors to recommend a basal/bolus insulin regimen. (While your diabetes care team will discuss this more in depth, you can think of basal insulin as background insulin and bolus insulin as mealtime insulin.) The basal/bolus regimen means giving a basal dose of a long-acting insulin and then a bolus dose of a rapid-acting insulin after meals. This way, the bolus dosage can accurately match the actual food eaten, taking out much of the guesswork and lowering the risk of hypoglycemia.

Because they are so small, infants require very small insulin adjustments, often less than one unit at a time. Your doctor may recommend that you use diluted insulin for your baby. If this is the case, either it will be diluted for you at the pharmacy or you should receive very specific information from your diabetes care team on the dilution process and the exact syringe to use. Insulin pumps are being used more commonly in babies and toddlers because they can deliver as little as one-tenth of a unit of insulin accurately.

Fifteen

I need to return to work soon. What is the ideal child care situation for my toddler?

There are a variety of options, but research and planning are essential. Family members may be the first people you turn to, but often it is necessary to arrange another child care option as well.

- Start your search by talking to your diabetes care team. They can recommend excellent community resources, including the local ADA and parent support groups.

- Nursing students, siblings of children with diabetes, or a teenager who has diabetes himself make great caregivers for toddlers with diabetes.

- Other parents of children with diabetes know firsthand about the challenges you face. Arrange to trade babysitting responsibilities with them for childcare needs and emotional support.

- Provide diabetes education for your child's caregivers. Simple explanations, specific guidelines, and "need to know" information should emphasize the fact that diabetes is unpredictable, especially in young children, making blood glucose checks very important. A thorough understanding of the symptoms and treatment of hypoglycemia is essential. Excellent resources are available on the website of the ADA (*www.diabetes.org*).

Sixteen

My son has a full-blown case of the "terrible twos." What can I do to handle the daily power struggles over blood glucose checks, insulin injections, and food?

Be flexible. Children at this age are trying to master their environment and make their own choices. Unfortunately, they can't quite understand the importance of their diabetes care routine and may be frightened by things such as blood glucose checks and injections. Added to the common struggle over food choices, this makes for a difficult situation. Try these methods:

- Give him a chance to make choices, such as where he'd like his injections, which finger to stick, and whether to have graham crackers or animal crackers for his snack. Make the choices reasonable and appropriate for his diabetes care regimen.
- Don't make not eating a major issue. Fighting at mealtime could increase your son's resistance and have long-lasting effects on his relationship with food. If he refuses your planned meal, calmly offer one or two alternatives. You and your diabetes care team may decide it's best to give a rapid-acting insulin injection after mealtime based on what your child actually eats.
- Praise your son whenever he cooperates with finger sticks, insulin injections, or meals. You might set up a star chart system where your son earns a star for each finger stick or shot. The stars can be "redeemed" for a trip to the playground, an extra bedtime story, or another favorite treat.

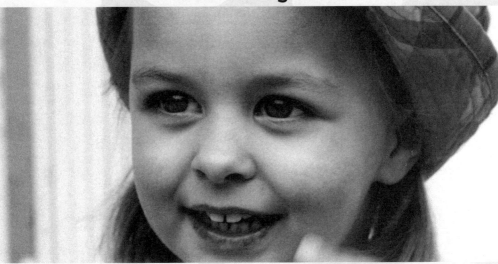

Chapter 3.
Preschool to Primary School:
ABC's of Management

Young children are beginning to gain a sense of self and an understanding that they are part of a community made up of family, friends, and school. They are aware of how people feel about them and want to please the adults in their lives—a welcome relief after life with a strong-willed toddler! They can begin to participate in their diabetes care and are active learners with vivid imaginations.

Seventeen

My 4 year old often refuses to eat. I know this can be dangerous, especially if we've already given her an insulin injection. Is there anything we can do?

Try defining the process. Forcing your child to eat will backfire in the long run, particularly if she associates eating with pressure or the desire to please others. The American Diabetes Association (ADA) book *Sweet Kids* offers several excellent suggestions to relieve some of the mealtime tension. The authors suggest sitting down together away from the table and developing mealtime "job descriptions."

The Parent's Job Description is to:
- Get the right foods on the table.
- Make family meals frequent, peaceful, and important.
- Eat what you want your children to eat.
- Set the rules and then stay in charge!

The Child's Job Description is to:
- Decide how much to eat of the available foods.
- Follow family rules for mealtime behavior.

Referring to these job descriptions will remove some of the strain from the relationship between you, your daughter, and food.

Eighteen

I've heard that "positive reinforcement" works well in this age-group. Any suggestions for staying upbeat in the face of our diabetes care duties?

Most four- to seven-year-old children want to please the adults in their lives, which makes positive reinforcement a good motivation for their cooperation with the daily diabetes care routine of eating right, taking medication, and monitoring blood glucose. Realistically, diabetes requires many extra tasks that can be difficult for a young child to tolerate or perform. Rewarding your child for cooperating won't spoil her anymore than having someone thank you for your efforts at work spoils you.

Catch your child being good. If you happen to notice that she's wearing her medical ID, say, "I see you're wearing your medical ID. I'm proud of you for doing the right thing to take care of your diabetes." Unexpected praise is a powerful reward. Remember to praise your child for her cooperation at other times with treats such as hugs, kisses, stickers, a walk in the park, or extra story time. It's best to avoid using food as a reward. Non-food items are a better choice because they won't affect blood glucose. Also, tying food to good behavior sends the wrong message that food is a reward.

Positive reinforcement is one of the strongest tools caregivers can use to encourage self-care behaviors in children with diabetes.

Nineteen

Between preschool and friends, our child is spending more time away from home. How should we share diabetes information with those that need to know?

Diabetes education for those responsible for your child is a must. Caregivers, coaches, teachers, and friends should know the basics about meals and snacks, blood glucose monitoring, medication, hypoglycemia, and hyperglycemia. A phone call or written instructions are always helpful. The ADA has several excellent resources on their website (*www.diabetes.org*) that parents can share, including a one-page information sheet for caregivers.

Sharing the care of your child with diabetes is one of the most difficult tasks for parents. The preschool and early school years are often the first time that a child with diabetes ventures outside of the safe borders of his home and, as a parent, you must begin to trust that others will keep him safe and take care of his diabetes properly.

The ultimate goal of raising a healthy child with diabetes is to help him learn how to best take care of himself. As he begins to step out into the world, the lessons that you teach him at home will make it easier for him to deal with the choices he faces everywhere, from school lunch to soccer games to sleepovers.

Twenty

We'd like our 7-year-old daughter to begin developing some independence in terms of her diabetes care. What should we be teaching her about diabetes at this age?

Start small. At this age, your daughter can help by doing simple diabetes care tasks, but you have the major responsibility for her diabetes management. Some concepts she should be learning include:

- Safety issues—importance of wearing medical identification
- Hypoglycemia—recognizing her symptoms; reporting them to the caregiver in charge; knowing when low blood glucose may occur; knowing what she needs to eat or drink when her glucose is low
- Hyperglycemia—knowing symptoms and actions to take
- Healthy eating—categorizing food into groups; recognizing sources of carbohydrate; portion sizes; basic concepts about the effects of food on blood glucose
- Physical activity—knowing the best types of physical activity for her; knowing that activity lowers blood glucose; importance of having rapidly absorbed carbohydrate available
- Monitoring—choosing a site for obtaining blood for glucose monitoring; completing a blood glucose check using a meter; writing down results of glucose checks in a log book
- Medication—knowing the time of day medication is to be taken; rotating insulin injection sites; safe storage of medication

Twenty
One

Our 6 year old doesn't seem to realize that skipping his snack will lead to low blood glucose later. Is this normal?

This is not out of the ordinary. Because of their developing imaginations and rich fantasy lives, preschool and early school-age children may have trouble linking their behavior to outcomes and consequences. Your son needs to learn to associate the behavior of skipping his snack with the result of hypoglycemia. This can be a difficult lesson to teach, particularly since you don't want him to actually experience the dangerous consequence of severe hypoglycemia. However, your goal is to gradually give him the full responsibility of snacking appropriately and on time.

Be sure to set out clear guidelines for snack time and what makes a healthy snack. Then involve your son in selecting his snack and choosing a way to carry it with him. Explain the sensation of low blood glucose to him, perhaps by reminding him of a time when he felt low and what treatment was required to make him feel better. Finally, you need to let him decide whether or not to eat his snack. Knowing that he may experience hypoglycemia if he skips it, you may only want to set up this situation when he is at home under your close supervision. He may experience anything from no symptoms of low blood glucose to severe hypoglycemia. Be ready with a treatment and a reminder explanation, but not an "I told you so." You should support your son's learning to manage his diabetes—and snacks—independently.

Twenty
Two

It seems impossible to guess what type of activity and appetite my 5-year-old son will have from day to day. How do we cope with this unpredictability?

By being flexible. Variations in activity and appetite from day to day are characteristic of the preschool to primary school-age group. How simple it would be if everything were in black and white. However, a large part of the charm of this age-group is the variety of color they add to our lives.

Your best strategy for dealing with unpredictability is flexibility– and frequent blood glucose checks! Overly rigid guidelines aren't necessary. Appetite and food intake are closely related to activity and energy needs. If your child has a busy day on the playground, you will most likely find that he eats a bit more to compensate for the calories he's burned. On the other hand, slower placed days mean a smaller need for food. Because children are growing, they may need extra food to promote growth and weight gain at certain times. Yet at other times, it seems like they just "stop eating."

The medication choices we now have available make it easier to deal with unpredictability as well. You may want to base your son's meal-related insulin dose on the amount of carbohydrate he actually ate, lowering his risk for low blood glucose. In this case, speak with your diabetes care team about giving his injection after meals rather than before.

Chapter 4.
School-Aged Children:
Adding Confidence, Subtracting Fear

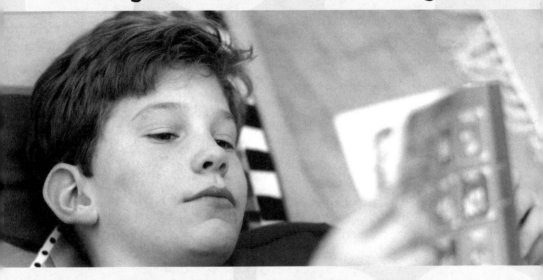

These children are developing athletic, cognitive, artistic, and social skills. They can be more actively involved in diabetes care tasks and take pride in being independent. Strengthening their self-esteem with respect to their peers is important to them.

Twenty Three

My 11-year-old daughter's pediatrician attributes her high blood glucose levels to a "growth spurt." How does growing affect blood glucose levels?

In a couple of ways. First, hormone changes in a growing body, especially during puberty, can have a dramatic impact on insulin needs. Growth hormones and the secretion of sex hormones contribute to insulin resistance, meaning the body doesn't use insulin as well. As the added insulin resistance occurs, blood glucose levels typically begin to rise. Also, a growing child's appetite may increase, leading to more food being eaten and a greater need for insulin. During growth spurts in children with type 1 diabetes, there is often a dramatic increase in insulin doses. In children with type 2 diabetes, modifications to their diabetes treatment plan may be necessary for optimal blood glucose control.

Twenty Four

My 9-year-old son doesn't want to go to school—he says his friends tease him about his diabetes, which makes him feel "different." How can I help?

Ask him. If your child is being teased, it is important to find out the details around each incident. Letting your son tell you how the teasing makes him feel will help you understand the effect it has on him. Because children with diabetes often feel different from their peers, there's a risk for social difficulties. Ideally, his diabetes care team includes a mental health professional, such as a psychologist or social worker, who can help him develop normal peer relationships. It may be helpful to discuss this issue with his physician, who can make any necessary referrals.

Encourage your son to attend school and participate in school activities and sports. These activities can help him understand that diabetes is not a barrier to these things. Activities that include other children with diabetes, such as diabetes camps, are also an excellent way to overcome the feeling of being different. Talk with the school counselor on a regular basis and plan ahead for school activities to assure your child's safety and participation.

Twenty Five

I found a bag of candy bars hidden in my son's dresser drawer. How should I deal with this?

Honestly. Let your son know that you came across the bag of candy bars in his room and ask him why he put them there. By asking him to tell you about the candy bars in the drawer, it will allow him to provide you his reasons. Once you have heard his reasons, then working with his diabetes treatment team may be helpful. For example, if he is truly "hiding" the candy bars, why is that? Sugary snacks do not need to be completely forbidden—an occasional candy bar can usually be worked into his diabetes meal plan with the help of a diabetes educator and registered dietitian. Teaching him how to do this may help him have an occasional treat while keeping good blood glucose control. It will also help him feel less deprived and show that you can be flexible and still take care of your diabetes.

Twenty Six

My 11 year old has a 3-year history of type 1 diabetes. Shouldn't he be able to perform blood glucose monitoring and insulin injections on his own?

Yes, but with supervision. School-aged children with diabetes can begin to assume more responsibility for tasks related to their diabetes. But they should be supervised and supported by caring adults who are knowledgeable about their individual diabetes treatment plan. Do not expect too much and try to avoid pushing your child into responsibilities too early. Also try to maintain perspective. The biggest chore asked of most children this age is taking out the trash or cleaning up after themselves. Being responsible for something as serious as proper blood glucose management is a big task.

Many children that master the day-to-day tasks quite well will still need a significant amount of help and guidance when it comes to troubleshooting and management decisions with regard to their diabetes. Several studies have shown that when children are relied on to manage their diabetes without proper adult supervision, the result is poorer glucose control. Until your child is older, the responsibility for diabetes care should be shared between you and your child.

Twenty Seven

My 8 year old was recently diagnosed with diabetes. Should I consider home schooling?

It depends. If you are considering home schooling simply because your child has diabetes, think again. There are no purely medical reasons to home school your child because of diabetes. Additionally, children with diabetes often feel different from other kids and can be at risk for problems socially. Home schooling your child may make these tendencies worse rather than better.

Still, home schooling can be a viable option for any child. According to the National Households Education Surveys (NHES) Program, parents may home school their children for a variety of reasons, but certain factors appear to have been more influential than others. Nearly two-thirds of home schooled students had parents who said their primary reason for home schooling was either concern about the environment of other schools or a desire to provide religious or moral instruction. It seems home schooling generally has more to do with values and philosophy than it does special medical requirements.

If you decide against home schooling, remember that sending a child with diabetes off to school requires every effort to make it a reality. Meet with your diabetes care team and work to make your child's diabetes care regimen fit for participation in school and school-related activities.

Chapter 5.
Adolescents:
Maturity Matters with Metabolism

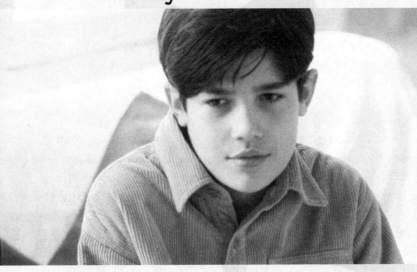

*In their early years, adolescents are experienc-
ing bodily changes, as well as developing a
strong sense of self-identity. As they mature,
they will further establish this self-identity after
high school and confront a variety of decisions
regarding further education, social issues, work,
and location.*

Twenty Eight

My teenage daughter says she is skipping insulin doses "to help with her weight." What should I do?

Seek professional help for your daughter that can show her that intentional or deliberate omission of insulin is dangerous. Many studies, which have found higher rates of both anorexia and bulimia in youth with type 1 diabetes, have described skipping insulin to lose weight as a type of eating disorder. How does skipping insulin cause weight loss? By not taking insulin, blood glucose levels can run high enough to eliminate glucose through the urine and lower the absorption of calories, which results in weight loss.

Adolescents with diabetes, especially girls, with this type of eating disorder are more likely to have recurrent hospitalizations and poor glucose control. Over time, the high blood glucose levels caused by skipping or reducing insulin places your daughter at much higher risk for the development of diabetes-related complications, such as retinopathy (eye disease), neuropathy (nerve disease), and nephropathy (kidney disease).

Twenty Nine

My 12-year-old son's pediatrician mentioned that he is "in the 96th percentile for weight" and is "insulin resistant." What does that mean?

First off, if your son is in the 96th percentile for weight, it means your son weighs the same or more than 96% of 12 year olds. Second, when your son's doctor says he is "insulin resistant," he's referring to a condition in which the body needs extra insulin to control blood glucose levels. For some reason (we're still not sure why), your son's body does not effectively use the insulin his pancreas produces. This can cause blood glucose levels to be higher than normal, leading to pre-diabetes or type 2 diabetes.

At this weight, your son is also at risk for other health conditions, including high blood pressure, high cholesterol and triglycerides, atherosclerosis, and other conditions. Your son's pediatrician should monitor him for these issues and work with you on a treatment plan for your son that includes working toward a healthy body weight and promotion of physical activity.

Thirty

My 16-year-old daughter said she was told that girls with diabetes couldn't have babies. Should I be concerned?

Yes. You should be concerned for at least two reasons. First, a female that has diabetes during her childbearing years (which is basically puberty through menopause) can become pregnant, unless there is another medical reason preventing pregnancy. In fact, women with diabetes can have normal, healthy children with proper planning and education. Why should this concern you? Because it is vitally important that there is good blood glucose control before pregnancy in order to prevent complications, including birth defects in the infant. Second, diabetes does not prevent pregnancy; therefore, proper birth control is necessary to prevent pregnancy whenever a female becomes sexually active.

Making sure your daughter is well educated about these issues is important. It may prevent endless worry if she plans to have children and help her understand that precautions should be taken to avoid pregnancy until she is ready.

Thirty One

I've noticed my son's voice has changed and he's grown facial hair. His recent A1C was 1.2% higher than the last check. Could these changes be affecting his A1C?

Yes. There is a strong link between puberty and insulin resistance, and the changes you describe (voice and facial hair) are common signs of maturity in boys. During puberty, there is an increased secretion of growth hormone, and this is likely the reason for the insulin resistance. Most children with type 2 diabetes are diagnosed around 13 years of age—the peak period of growth and maturity in puberty. For those with type 1 diabetes, insulin doses will probably need to be increased substantially during puberty.

It is important to avoid getting frustrated during this difficult time, both in a child's life and in his or her diabetes treatment. Blood glucose levels can often be erratic. However, your child's diabetes treatment plan needs to be monitored and modified as necessary to help aim for the best possible blood glucose control.

Thirty
Two

My daughter seems to consistently have high blood glucose levels at the start of her menstrual period. Why is that?

Blood glucose levels are usually higher around the time of menstruation. Some women may notice the rise in blood glucose just before and others will see it during their menstrual period. The higher blood glucose levels typically last about 3-5 days. During menstruation, a natural release of hormones causes the body to become more resistant to insulin, whether a person has diabetes or not. During this period of high blood glucose levels, most women adjust their treatment plan with more insulin to handle the higher glucose levels. As the release of hormones decreases, however, blood glucose levels may drop, sometimes rapidly. In some cases, the combination of dropping hormones and extra insulin can lead to hypoglycemia (low blood glucose). If hypoglycemia occurs, it is important to treat it promptly. Work with your diabetes treatment team to recognize and accommodate patterns of both high as well as low blood glucose levels that are related to the menstrual cycle.

Thirty Three

My 13-year-old daughter's pediatrician is referring her to an endocrinologist for "PCOS and insulin resistance." Is this really necessary?

Yes. Polycystic ovarian syndrome (PCOS) is a female endocrine disorder marked by high levels of male hormones and is linked to a 40% decrease in insulin sensitivity and problems in the beta cells that make insulin. Unfortunately, PCOS is being recognized more and more in adolescent females. Common symptoms of PCOS include:

- Irregular menstrual cycles
- Acne
- Acanthosis nigricans (dark patches of skin, usually on the neck, groin, or underarms; see page 97)
- Hirsutism (growth of coarse body hair in a male pattern, such as on the face and chest)

Seeing an endocrinologist early can help your daughter develop a treatment plan that is right for her, as well as monitor her risk for additional health-related issues. It is important to note that about 40% of women with PCOS develop pre-diabetes or type 2 diabetes.

Chapter 6.
Healthy Eating for Healthy Kids

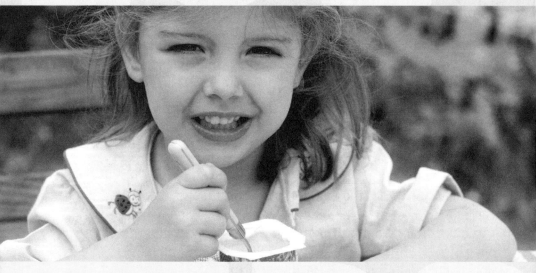

*C*hildren with diabetes have the same nutri-tional needs as children without diabetes. *Healthy eating, balanced with physical activity and medication management, is essential for normal growth and development, as well as good blood glucose control.*

Thirty Four

I thought people with diabetes couldn't have sugar, but our dietitian told us just to watch carbohydrates. Which is more important, sugar or carbohydrates?

The answer, in a way, is "both." Carbohydrate is the body's main fuel source and the nutrient that most directly affects blood glucose. Sugar is just one type of carbohydrate food, as are grains, beans, starchy vegetables, fruit, milk and yogurt, and sweets.

People with diabetes used to be told to avoid sugar. However, research has shown that sugar from candy, for example, doesn't necessarily raise blood glucose faster or higher than a starchy food such as potatoes or rice. While the type of carbohydrate does influence blood glucose levels, the amount of carbohydrate should be of more concern. Carbohydrate needs vary based on age and activity level and can range from 195 grams per day for a preschool child up to 300 grams per day for an adolescent boy. Results from blood glucose monitoring help determine the ideal meal plan.

Sugar is not "off limits" if it is included as part of, not in addition to, the total carbohydrate allowance for the day. However, it's wise to encourage healthier carbohydrate choices. In addition to being bad for the teeth, sugary foods are often "empty calories" (lots of calories, few vitamins and minerals) and filled with fat as well. Overall good nutrition along with good blood glucose control is the most important goal.

Thirty Five

We don't believe in eating between meals. Does my 9-year-old son with diabetes really need snacks?

Probably. Most children, even those without diabetes, need snacks between meals to nip hunger in the bud and to provide calories for growth and development. Snacks may be even more important for children with diabetes to prevent hypoglycemia (low blood glucose) between meals and during exercise. For example, if your son is on a fixed insulin dose, his meals and snacks need to match the peak of his insulin action to prevent hypoglycemia. If he is on a flexible insulin dose, also known as the basal-bolus approach, he may not need a snack to match the peak of his insulin since he will be taking a bolus dose of insulin when he chooses to eat. In both cases, however, a snack may be required during physical activity.

A child's appetite, growth phase, and physical activity will determine the number of snacks to include each day. In general, a child less than 6 years of age may need three snacks if there are more than 4 or 5 hours between meals. Older children need midafternoon and bedtime snacks. However, a child with type 2 diabetes who is taking no diabetes medication should only eat when truly hungry and stop when he is full.

Snacks generally do not lead to weight gain unless they are excessive amounts of poor nutritional choices, such as snack pastries and processed foods. Snack time is a great time to include fruits, vegetables, and dairy products in your child's meal plan. Some snack suggestions include: cereal and low-fat milk, fruit and low-fat cheddar cheese, half a peanut butter sandwich, or crackers and string cheese.

Thirty Six

My daughter has type 2 diabetes and wants to lose weight. How can she accomplish this goal?

By making lifestyle changes such as healthy eating and physical activity. These changes will help keep blood glucose as close to target range as possible and improve your daughter's overall health. Some tips for weight loss in children:

- Make movement fun! Encourage your daughter to enjoy activity, particularly school sports, dance lessons, or active games.
- Limit screen time. Overweight children often spend hours in front of the computer, watching television, or playing video games. Have your daughter take activity breaks for 10 minutes for every half hour of screen time.
- Become an aware eater. Encourage your daughter to stop eating unconsciously, out of boredom, or while studying or watching TV. If she thinks before she eats and eats slowly, she will better recognize being full and will avoid overeating.
- Keep an eye on portion size. Reducing portion sizes is the easiest way to cut calories without banishing favorite foods. Have your daughter leave a little food on her plate at every meal.
- Find the fat. The fat in high-fat foods such as fries, chips, and full-fat dairy products has twice as many calories per serving as proteins and carbohydrates.
- Skip the sugar. Sugar is generally an empty-calorie, low-nutrition food. Substitute water for sugared beverages.

Thirty Seven

Why are portion sizes so important? Do we have to weigh and measure everything our son eats?

Whether your child has type 1 or type 2 diabetes, portion sizes are extremely important to help you know how many grams of carbohydrate or calories he eats. Don't worry though; you won't need to measure every morsel of food for the rest of your son's life. Start by measuring food and beverages during the first few weeks after diagnosis in order to imprint a mental picture of proper serving sizes in your mind's eye. Then double-check yourself occasionally to prevent a slip into "portion distortion." Prepackaged and labeled foods such as granola bars or packs of cheese crackers are one way of knowing exactly what a serving of food contains. Another way to size up your servings is to compare them to familiar items:

- A small baked potato is about the size of a computer mouse.
- A clenched fist is about the size of a one-cup serving of pasta, rice, fruit, or vegetable.
- Half a tennis ball is about the size of 1/2 cup of vegetables or fruit. A one-cup serving of broccoli is the size of a light bulb.
- Three ounces of meat, poultry, or fish is about the size of a deck of playing cards, a woman's palm, or a computer mouse.
- One ounce of cheese is about the size of an adult thumb or four dice.
- Your thumb is about the size of one tablespoon; the tip of your thumb is about one teaspoon.

Thirty Eight

There is so much information on food labels! What should we be looking at? Sugar? Carbohydrate? Fat? Calories?

The Nutrition Facts label contains a lot of information—almost too much it can seem! Start by focusing on the total carbohydrate and calories of a single serving of the food. This will help you determine if the food fits into a meal plan and how to match insulin dose to the food. Some key areas:

Serving size—There is often more than one serving in a packaged food, and the serving size on the label may be different than the serving size you're used to eating.

Total carbohydrate—If you're tracking carbohydrate servings, divide the total carbohydrate listed by 15 to get the number of carbohydrate servings.

Calories—Be careful: many fat-free and sugar-free foods can still be high in calories.

Fiber—If a serving has more than 5 grams of fiber, subtract the amount of fiber from the total carbohydrate.

Sugar alcohol—If there are more than 10 grams of sugar alcohol, subtract 1/2 the grams of sugar alcohol from the total carbohydrate.

Nutrition Facts

Serving Size 1 cup (228g)
Servings Per Container 2

Amount Per Serving

Calories 260   Calories from Fat 120

		% Daily Value*
Total Fat 13g		**20%**
Saturated Fat 5g		**25%**
Trans Fat 2g		
Cholesterol 30mg		**10%**
Sodium 660mg		**28%**
Total Carbohydrate 31g		**10%**
Dietary Fiber 0g		**0%**
Sugars 5g		
Protein 5g		

Vitamin A 4%	•	Vitamin C 2%
Calcium 15%	•	Iron 4%

* Percent Daily Values are based on a 2,000 calorie diet. Your Daily Values may be higher or lower depending on your calorie needs.

	Calories:	2,000	2,500
Total Fat	Less than	65g	80g
Sat Fat	Less than	20g	25g
Cholesterol	Less than	300mg	300mg
Sodium	Less than	2,400mg	2,400mg
Total Carbohydrate		300g	375g
Dietary Fiber		25g	30g

Calories per gram:
Fat 9   •   Carbohydrate 4   •   Protein 4

Thirty Nine

Our family has always enjoyed eating out on the weekends. Can we still enjoy that family tradition?

Yes. Eating out healthfully can be a challenge for anyone, but diabetes should not get in the way of fun family traditions. Here are a few tips for restaurant dining:

- Be especially aware of huge portions that may contain excess amounts of calories, carbohydrate, fat, and sodium.
- Do some research. Chain and fast food restaurants often have websites or information sheets with the exact nutrient and exchange information of each item. The American Diabetes Association's *Guide to Healthy Restaurant Eating* is also an excellent resource.
- Order high-fat dressings, sauces, and gravy on the side.
- Choose low-fat methods of food preparation such as grilled, broiled, roasted, baked, or steamed.
- Skip super sizing and substitute a salad with low-fat dressing for French fries.
- Share dessert and choose water or low-fat milk instead of regular soft drinks.
- Reduce the risk of hypoglycemia from a delayed meal by injecting the bolus dose as the food arrives.
- Keep in mind that high-fat meals such as pizza or Mexican food can delay stomach emptying, leading to high blood glucose levels for up to 6–8 hours after eating.

Forty

I know sugar isn't completely "off limits." But is it better for my daughter to have sugar-free foods?

It depends. Sugar is just one form of carbohydrate. Sugar doesn't necessarily raise blood glucose faster or higher than other forms of carbohydrate, but because sweets are bad for the teeth and sweet treats are often high in fat and low in vitamins and minerals, it's best to save them for an occasional indulgence. And they should always be included in the carbohydrate content of the meal plan.

If you'd like to use sugar-free foods, read labels carefully. Check the total carbohydrate content on the food label. If a nutritive sweetener has been used, a food labeled as "sugar-free" may not be calorie or carbohydrate free. Sugar alcohols (also known as polyols) such as sorbitol and xylitol provide approximately 2 calories per gram as well as being a source of carbohydrate.

Non-nutritive sweeteners provide a sweet taste without calories or carbohydrate. The Food and Drug Administration (FDA) has approved five non-nutritive sweeteners as safe for use within the FDA Acceptable Daily Intake: saccharin (Sweet 'N Low, Sugar Twin), aspartame (NutraSweet, NatraTaste), sucralose (Splenda), acesulfame potassium (SweetOne and Sunette), and neotame.

Forty One

Do children with diabetes need special vitamins?

Not necessarily. Children with diabetes have the same nutrient requirements as those without diabetes. In general, children in the United States don't eat the recommended amounts of fruits and vegetables. However, research shows that children with diabetes may be doing somewhat better than their peers in proper intake of calories, vitamins, and minerals.

The food pyramid is a good guideline to follow to make sure your child is getting the proper amounts of vitamins and minerals from a variety of healthful foods. Based on an 1800-calorie diet, a healthy, complete meal plan for the day contains:

- 6 ounces of grains, with at least half being whole grains
- 2 1/2 cups of vegetables
- 1 1/2 cups of fruit
- 2–3 cups of low-fat milk
- 5 ounces of lean protein

Your child probably does not need a vitamin supplement if he is eating this way on a daily basis. Visit the newly updated USDA website *www.mypyramid.gov* for more information on vitamins and minerals for your child.

Forty Two

I'm not sure how much my 8 year old should eat. If his blood sugar is high, should we have him skip his snacks? If it's low, should we force him to eat more?

Not usually. To manage diabetes, children need the right amount of food as well as the correct amount of insulin at the proper time. Withholding food or having your child eat when he's not hungry are not good ways to control blood glucose in the long run. There are exceptions, such as treating hypoglycemia. Normally, though, appetite adjusts to calorie needs without much outside control. Your child's hunger is the best guide to how much food he should eat. But keep in mind that inactivity and super size portions may confuse this internal regulation. Keep checking his blood glucose control and pay attention to two other factors:

- **Hunger** reflects the need for energy and varies from day to day based on activity level and growth stage.
- **Growth** is a long-term measure of nutritional needs being met, which can be plotted on a pediatric growth chart at physician visits. If your child is not staying on his growth curve or if his height and weight percentiles are out of proportion, your health care team may need to take a closer look at his eating, activity level, diabetes management, and general health.

Good metabolic control is essential for normal growth and development. However, you should not withhold food or force a child to eat when he's not hungry in an effort to control blood glucose.

Forty Three

My daughter has a hard time sticking to her meal plan, especially if other kids tease her about diabetes. How can we help her be more confident in her food choices?

Developing social skills and enlisting the support of her friends will help your daughter become more confident with her food choices. Your daughter faces many challenges when dealing with diabetes and food choices away from home, particularly if she is afraid of being seen as different or having more restrictions than her friends.

Helping your daughter's friends learn more about diabetes by inviting them home for a healthy cooking session or casually talking with them about her food plan may enlist their support and encouragement and stop the teasing. Your daughter may want to do a "show and tell" at school about healthy foods for diabetes or ask your diabetes nutrition educator to do it for or with her. If your daughter develops effective social skills, such as learning to deal with peer pressure, teasing, and misconceptions about diabetes, it will help her become more confident about her food choices and diabetes management in general.

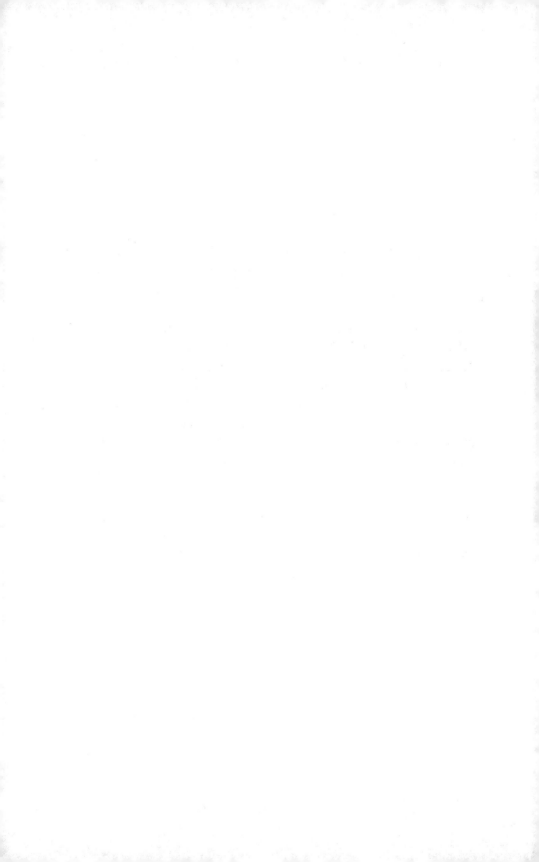

Chapter 7.
The Art and Science of Medication Management

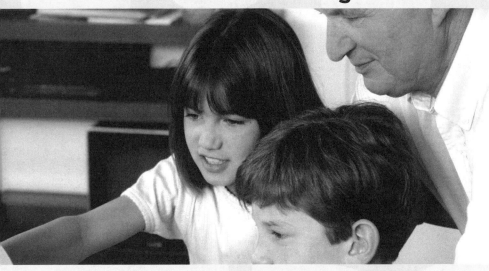

*C*hildren with type 1 diabetes require insulin to maintain optimal glucose control. In type 2 diabetes, the aim of pharmacological therapy is to decrease insulin resistance, increase insulin secretion, or slow post-meal glucose absorption. Use of oral anti-hyperglycemic agents and/or insulin is indicated when needed to meet blood glucose targets.

Forty Four

Can insulin be given any other way besides an injection?

Not yet for children. Inhalable insulin is now on the market for adults with type 1 and type 2 diabetes, but it's not currently approved for use in kids. Other than in a medical setting, the only method approved by the Food and Drug Administration (FDA) for children in the U.S. is to inject insulin into the fatty tissue just below the skin, usually in the abdomen, arms, buttocks, or thighs.

There are various devices that can be used to accomplish an insulin injection. A syringe can be used to pull insulin from a vial and then inject it into the body. Insulin pens are another insulin delivery method, with both reusable and disposable models available. Reusable insulin pens and devices use cartridges of insulin that can be replaced as needed. Disposable pens and devices are prefilled with insulin and then thrown away once they're empty. Insulin pumps, which are small, computerized, mechanical devices about the size of a pager, are also used to infuse insulin. Insulin pumps deliver insulin by pumping rapid- or short-acting insulin through plastic tubing to a small catheter, or needle, that is inserted into the fat layer under the skin and taped in place. The infusion set is usually changed about every 48 hours. Another less commonly used option is a jet injector, which sends a fine spray of insulin through the skin using a high-pressure air mechanism instead of a needle.

Regardless of the type of method used to administer insulin, it is important to work with the diabetes treatment team to determine the best option and provide proper education and training for success.

Forty Five

I don't understand "basal" versus "bolus" insulin. What's the difference?

Basal insulin is background insulin and bolus insulin is mealtime insulin. But what does this mean?

The body needs a small amount of background insulin at all times to keep blood glucose levels controlled between meals and overnight. Individuals who do not have diabetes (or who do have diabetes but whose pancreas still produces insulin) constantly secrete this small amount of so-called background, or basal, insulin. In an individual with diabetes whose pancreas does not produce insulin (or does not produce enough), this basal insulin needs to come from injecting intermediate- or long-acting insulin or by using an insulin pump that is programmed to continuously deliver small pulses of short- or rapid-acting insulin.

At mealtimes, blood glucose levels rise as carbohydrates are digested and enter the bloodstream as glucose. A healthy pancreas responds by releasing a burst of insulin so that the amount of insulin released matches the rise in blood glucose. Individuals with diabetes who use insulin can match the pancreas's action by injecting a dose of short- or rapid-acting insulin before the meal or by taking a dose with an insulin pump, which acts as a bolus to cover the amount of carbohydrate that is eaten in the meal, or in some cases a snack. Bolus doses of insulin can also be taken to correct high blood glucose. These doses are also referred to as correction doses.

Forty
Six

My 3-year-old child won't eat her lunch. Should I still give her rapid-acting insulin?

Not if she won't eat anything at all. Her physician may recommend waiting until after she actually eats to give the insulin. Rapid-acting insulin (such as aspart, lispro, and glulisine) is usually taken with food to cover the nutrients, particularly carbohydrate, eaten in the meal. However, toddlers can make this process a little more difficult to manage. If your child is a picky eater or eats different amounts from meal to meal, giving insulin before she eats can pose the risk of hypoglycemia (low blood glucose). Studies have shown that it's possible to give rapid-acting insulin after meals in very young children, such as your daughter. Doing this will allow you to more accurately figure out the dose for your picky eater, with the goal of matching the actual food intake and insulin more closely. For more information, consult with a registered dietitian who has experience in pediatric nutrition and diabetes.

Forty Seven

Is there any advantage for my son to use an insulin pen versus an insulin syringe?

Maybe. An insulin pen can be useful with intensive insulin therapy, especially if your son takes several injections away from home. With a pen, there's no need to draw up insulin into the syringe because the pen has an insulin reservoir and the desired dose is simply dialed in. After injecting the needle into the fatty tissue in the proper site, the insulin is delivered by pushing the dose knob until it stops. Insulin pens also look less clinical and are more convenient to carry in a pocket, purse, or bag. The syringe and pen are still just delivery devices, so the timing, onset, peak, and duration of the specific type of insulin used should not vary between the two delivery methods. Depending on his age, it would probably be best to ask your son for input when choosing to use an insulin pen versus an insulin syringe.

Forty Eight

My son's endocrinologist prescribed a medication called "glucagon" for treatment of hypoglycemia. Is this really necessary?

Yes, in severe cases. Glucagon is a hormone that is normally produced by the pancreas and comes in a kit that can be used in an emergency situation related to hypoglycemia (such as when a person is unconscious or is unable to swallow any oral treatment). Glucagon is injected, usually in an area of fatty tissue, such as the back of the arms. Once injected, the hormone causes the liver to release glucose into the bloodstream, raising the blood glucose level.

Glucagon needs to be given by a designated person properly trained to give the injection, such as a family member or friend. Special precautions are necessary to assure the injection is given correctly and that the person receiving the injection is positioned properly prior to receiving the drug. Appropriate training in the use of glucagon by the diabetes educator, doctor, and/or pharmacist is encouraged.

Forty Nine

Can my daughter take pills for her diabetes?

It depends on the type of diabetes. If your daughter has type 1 diabetes, then the answer is no. Type 1 diabetes is a disorder that results from the destruction of the insulin-producing beta cells in the pancreas. Because your daughter can no longer produce insulin on her own, she will need to take outside insulin to metabolize glucose. Unfortunately, insulin is destroyed by the acids in the stomach, so taking it by pill is not an option. Instead, it must be injected, infused, or, possibly in the near future, inhaled.

If your daughter has type 2 diabetes, then the answer is maybe. Type 2 diabetes is a disorder where the body either makes too little insulin or doesn't use it efficiently (or both). The initial treatment for type 2 diabetes is typically meal planning and exercise designed for optimal blood glucose control. If glucose targets are not met, your doctor may then suggest oral diabetes medications. Currently, the only medication approved by the Federal Drug Administration (FDA) for use in children is metformin. In some cases, insulin may be the drug of choice for children with type 2 diabetes.

Fifty

Our daughter was diagnosed with type 1 about a month ago and she's taking much less insulin than when she was diagnosed. Is there a chance she won't need insulin?

Not likely. Several weeks after starting insulin therapy, it's common for a newly diagnosed child with diabetes to enter what is called the "honeymoon" phase. During the honeymoon phase, the remaining beta cells in your daughter's pancreas (the beta cells usually aren't destroyed all at once) actually increase insulin production, which means your daughter will need much less insulin than she did right after being diagnosed. It is important to realize that the beta cells are still being destroyed during the honeymoon phase. Continue monitoring blood glucose levels. The honeymoon phase will come to an end and you'll need to adjust insulin doses to cover the continued loss of insulin-producing beta cells.

Fifty
One

Is an insulin pump a good idea for my toddler?

Maybe. More and more children with diabetes are turning to con-
tinuous subcutaneous insulin infusion (CSII), or insulin pump
therapy. There is no "best" age to initiate pump therapy; the use of
pump therapy is determined by the individual needs of the child and
family. However, there are fewer young children and toddlers on
pumps than pre-adolescents and adolescents. Experience with pump
therapy indicates that candidates for insulin pump therapy must:

- Be strongly motivated to improve glucose control
- Be willing to work with their health care provider
- Assume much of the responsibility for day-to-day care
- Understand and demonstrate the use of an insulin pump
- Be willing and able to frequently self-monitor blood glucose
- Know how to use the data from self-monitoring

In a toddler's case, the parents or guardian would be responsible for
most of the pump management. Insulin pumps generally offer flexibility with insulin dosing, as well as safety features that prevent the toddler from pushing the buttons that activate the pump. Many parents
like that there are less needle sticks with insulin pump therapy, as
opposed to multiple daily insulin injections. To learn more about this
option, talk with a physician and a diabetes educator who have experience with insulin pump therapy.

Fifty Two

My daughter is 18 and has had type 1 diabetes for 10 years. Her physician wants to put her on a drug called an "ACE inhibitor." Is this for diabetes?

Not exactly. An angiotensin-converting enzyme (ACE) inhibitor is a drug commonly used to treat hypertension (high blood pressure). If your daughter does not have high blood pressure, then her physician is likely prescribing the medication because microalbuminuria, trace amounts of protein in the urine, has been detected. Microalbuminuria is a sign of early nephropathy (kidney disease), but at a stage when it may be reversible with careful blood glucose and blood pressure control. Even if your daughter does not have high blood pressure, therapy with an ACE inhibitor can reverse the excretion of albumin by the kidneys or delay further progression of kidney disease, a complication that can occur from poorly controlled diabetes.

Chapter 8.
Child's Play:
Physical Activity and Exercise

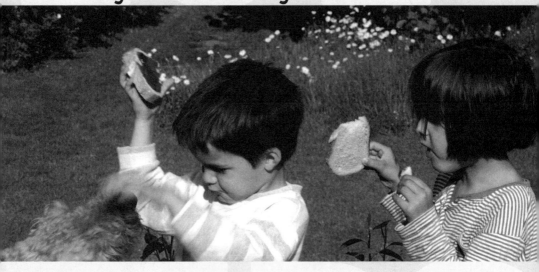

*P*hysical activity, as well as regular, planned exercise, provides emotional, social, and health benefits to all children. Lower blood glucose levels are an additional bonus for children with diabetes. Planning ahead for the risks, symptoms, and treatment of hypoglycemia will allow physical activity to be a safe and enjoyable part of your child's life.

Fifty
Three

My son was just diagnosed with type 2 diabetes. How can I get him interested in exercise?

There are a variety of ways. Your son doesn't have to be a competitive athlete to reap the benefits of physical activity; every child has his own natural activity level. The challenge is to identify the activities he enjoys and to encourage him to be active enough to stay healthy and control his weight as part of managing his type 2 diabetes.

Start slowly and keep it simple. Even 20 minutes a day can improve his health, lower his blood glucose, and give him more energy. Perhaps he'll need to begin with only 5 minutes of activity a day and increase the amount each week. A few suggestions:

- Walk the family dog.
- Take the stairs instead of the elevator or escalator.
- Ride bikes with friends.
- Listen to music or a book on tape while walking in the neighborhood or mall.
- Play catch.
- Enjoy old-fashioned games such as jump rope, hula-hoop, hopscotch, or foursquare.
- Play some favorite music and dance, dance, dance!

Managing type 2 diabetes in children requires family support and participation in the treatment plan. Make time to join him in his active pursuits, which will benefit your health and well-being, too!

Fifty
Four

Why is physical activity so important for a child with diabetes?

Because physical activity plays an important role in the treatment of a child with diabetes. Benefits of physical activity include:

- Greater sense of well-being, self-esteem, and self-confidence
- Help with weight control
- Improved physical fitness
- Increased muscle strength
- Improved cardiovascular fitness, including slower pulse and lower blood pressure
- Improved lipid profile
- Increased insulin sensitivity
- Decreased insulin resistance
- Potentially overall lower blood glucose levels

Children who take insulin and exercise regularly usually need less insulin than other children with diabetes. For overweight or obese children with diabetes, physical activity is a major tool for weight management.

As a parent, you can set a positive example by leading an active lifestyle yourself and making physical activity part of your family's daily routine. Provide opportunities for your child to be active by playing with him. Be positive about the physical activities in which your child participates and encourage him as he expresses interest in new activities.

Fifty Five

Should my 15-year-old daughter check her blood glucose while she's exercising?

Yes. The American Diabetes Association recommends checking blood glucose before and at the end of exercise and hourly during exercise if it's prolonged and strenuous. It's safest to keep blood glucose between 100 and 150 mg/dl during physical activity. General guidelines for blood glucose management during exercise include:

- If blood glucose is less than 150 mg/dl before exercise, have your daughter eat a small snack before exercising. A general guideline is that 15-30 grams of carbohydrate is needed for each 30-60 minutes of physical activity. Younger children with a smaller body mass may only need 5-10 grams of carbohydrate for each 30 minutes of physical activity.
- If blood glucose is in the 150-250 mg/dl range, it's generally safe to begin exercising. This level allows a safe margin for the drop in blood glucose usually associated with physical activity.
- If blood glucose is higher than 250 mg/dl, your daughter should not begin exercising without checking her urine for ketones and, if they are present, taking insulin to prevent ketoacidosis and higher blood glucose.

Since a variety of factors may influence blood glucose levels, such as training sessions that run long or anxiety prior to a big game, it's important to check periodically (during halftime or a timeout) and immediately if symptoms of low blood glucose occur.

Fifty Six

I've heard it is dangerous for a child with diabetes to exercise if his or her blood glucose is over 240 mg/dl. What precautions should we take?

If your child's blood glucose is over 240 mg/dl (or the level your diabetes team determines), check urine for ketones. Because ketones are the by-product of fat metabolism, their presence is a sign your child is burning fat instead of glucose for energy. If ketones are present, your child shouldn't exercise until they are gone. You may need to contact your physician to determine the exact steps to take, but generally, extra insulin and fluids are required to remove ketones from the body.

Surprisingly, exercise can raise blood glucose if there's not enough insulin present in your child's system to move the existing glucose into the cells for energy. In the situation of high blood glucose with ketones present, the ketones are a sign that the body does not have enough insulin. This lack of insulin can lead to diabetic ketoacidosis, a serious situation in which the blood can turn acidic, causing coma and death if left untreated.

If your child's blood glucose before exercise is over 300 mg/dl, it's best to take insulin and delay exercise until blood glucose levels return to target range, whether or not ketones are present.

Fifty
Seven

Sometimes my daughter's blood glucose falls very low during the night after she's had a particularly active day. Why would that happen hours later?

Because blood glucose levels can continue to fall long after your daughter has finished exercising. Physical activity and exercise lowers blood glucose and draws on stored glucose (glycogen) from the liver and muscles. If glycogen is not replaced by eating carbohydrates within 30 minutes after exercise, it can lead to delayed hypoglycemia 1-6 hours or even up to 24 hours after exercise has stopped. Replacing the glycogen by eating carbohydrate lowers the risk of hypoglycemia and also prepares your daughter's body for the next bout of exercise. Often, exercise in the late afternoon or evening can increase the chance of hypoglycemia during the night.

Be especially alert to preventing hypoglycemia after exercise on a particularly active day. Check your daughter's blood glucose before bedtime and be sure she has a bedtime snack. If you daughter uses an insulin pump, you may need to decrease the basal rate during exercise and perhaps overnight since hypoglycemia after exercise often occurs in the middle of the night.

Fifty Eight

Physical activity always lowers my son's blood glucose. Should we decrease his insulin or have him eat more carbohydrate before he exercises?

It depends on your son's situation. If your child is only participating in light activity or exercising less than 1 hour, it may be easier to add food rather than adjust insulin. If your child is overweight, it may be better to lower his insulin dose rather than add extra calories and carbohydrate. In some cases, a combination of adjusting both insulin and food works best.

If you'd rather adjust food, check your son's blood glucose before and at the end of exercise and at hourly intervals if he's participating in a prolonged strenuous activity. If blood glucose is less than 150 mg/dl before exercise, take some precautions before being active. If you'd like to adjust his food rather than his insulin, have him eat a small snack. A general guideline is that 15-30 grams of carbohydrate is needed for each 30-60 minutes of physical activity. Younger children with smaller bodies may only need 5-10 grams of carbohydrate for each 30 minutes of physical activity. During activity, 15 grams of carbohydrate in the form of readily absorbed sugar should be given if at any time blood glucose drops lower than 100 mg/dl.

If you'd like to adjust insulin, it's best to decrease the insulin that is most active during the exercise session by 30-50% to start, particularly if exercise will last longer than 30-60 minutes. You can lower long-acting, basal insulin by 10-20%, but never eliminate it entirely. If your son is on an insulin pump, lower his basal rate for the 4-6 hours after exercise by 50% to avoid post-exercise hypoglycemia.

Work with the diabetes care team to develop a plan that meets your son's needs.

Fifty
Nine

How should we choose a sports drink for our child with diabetes? Shouldn't she only be drinking sugar-free fluids?

Not necessarily. Children with diabetes may need extra water and carbohydrate to replace losses from exercise, particularly if they are active for longer than 60-90 minutes. Choose your daughter's beverage carefully to replenish fluid losses during activity.

- Cool, plain water is best for fluid replacement before, during, and after short-term exercise that lasts no longer than 60-90 minutes. Unless the exercise is especially intense, the electrolytes and carbohydrate found in sports drinks are probably not necessary.

- Research has found that flavored beverages containing sodium, such as sports drinks, may be preferable, especially if the taste encourages the child to drink more.

- Avoid caffeine-containing beverages, such as colas or tea, because of their mild diuretic effect.

- Read sports beverage labels carefully. A 6-8% carbohydrate solution empties from the stomach just like water, but will provide some extra carbohydrate. If the carbohydrate content is over 10%, such as fruit juice, it will empty more slowly from the stomach. Dilute fruit juices with water for faster absorption. Avoid beverages with a high concentration of carbohydrate, such as energy drinks; they can cause gastric distress including cramps and diarrhea, nausea, and bloating.

Chapter 9.
Monitoring:
Checking Up on Blood Glucose Control

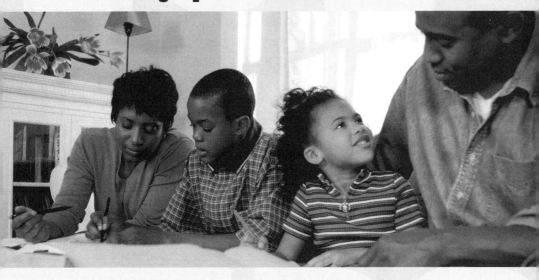

*S*elf-monitoring of blood glucose allows children with diabetes and their families to measure blood glucose levels rapidly and accurately. Self-monitoring is necessary to achieve optimal glucose control. There is a strong correlation between frequency of monitoring and glucose control.

Sixty

My daughter has type 1 diabetes. What should her blood glucose level be?

It will likely depend on her age along with other individual consider- ations. The following goals may be appropriate for kids with type 1 diabetes (see table below). However, get input from your diabetes care team to determine what the best target blood glucose levels are for her. Higher blood glucose targets may be necessary if your daughter has frequent hypoglycemia (low blood glucose) or episodes of hypo- glycemia where she does not recognize it (hypoglycemia unawareness). If there is a difference in self-blood glucose monitoring results and the laboratory analysis of her A1C (an 8- to 12-week blood glucose average), her doctor may recommend checking glucose levels 1-2 hours after the beginning of a meal to provide some extra insight.

Values by Age	Before Meals	Bedtime/ Overnight	A1C	Rationale
Toddlers & pre- schoolers (<6 yrs)	100-180 mg/dl	110-200 mg/dl	<8.5% (but >7.5%)	High risk & vulnerable to hypoglycemia
School age (6-12 yrs)	90-180 mg/dl	100-180 mg/dl	<8%	Risk of hypo- glycemia & relatively low risk of compli- cations
Adolescents (13-19 yrs)	90-130 mg/dl	90-150 mg/dl	<7.5%*	Developmental & psychologi- cal issues

*A lower goal (<7.0%) is reasonable if it can be achieved without excessive hypoglycemia.

Adapted from: Care of Children and Adolescents with Type 1 Diabetes, Table 4–Plasma blood glucose and A1C goals for type 1 diabetes by age group. *Diabetes Care*, Vol. 28, No. 1, Jan. 2005, p. 193.

Sixty One

What are the target blood glucose ranges for kids with type 2 diabetes?

Target blood glucose levels for kids with type 2 diabetes are typically the same as the goals for adults with type 2 diabetes.

Before meals	After meals (peak)	A1C
90–130 mg/dl	<180 mg/dl	<7.0%

Adapted from: Standards of Medical Care, Table 6—Summary of recommendations for adults with diabetes. *Diabetes Care*, Jan. 2006, Vol. 29, Suppl. 1, p. S10.

Because children with type 2 diabetes run a much lower risk for hypoglycemia with their treatment plans as compared to children with type 1 diabetes, the adult blood glucose targets may be recommended. However, if the child or adolescent taking an oral medication has the potential for hypoglycemia or if insulin is being used with treatment, then these goals may need to be modified. If there is a difference in self-blood glucose monitoring results and the laboratory analysis of A1C (an 8- to 12-week blood glucose average), the diabetes care team may recommend checking glucose levels 1–2 hours after the beginning of a meal to provide some additional insight. It is necessary to work with your diabetes care team to determine the blood glucose levels that are the best and safest for your child.

Sixty Two

What is an A1C?

An A1C (hemoglobin A1c) is a blood test that gives an estimate of average blood glucose levels over an 8- to 12-week period. The A1C is an important part of diabetes management. By giving a general average of blood glucose levels over an extended period of time, it gives a good snapshot of your child's blood glucose management in general, as opposed to a blood glucose monitor, which tells you where levels are at that instant. It can also be useful in predicting the risk for diabetes-related complications.

The A1C test is usually recommended every 3 months in kids with diabetes. Although equipment for A1C testing at home is available, the blood test is usually performed by a member of your child's health team and determined by laboratory analysis. Recommendations for A1C levels in kids with diabetes may vary depending on their age and the type of diabetes (see the tables on pages 74 and 75 for recommendations). Discuss the goal for your child's A1C with his or her diabetes care team.

Sixty Three

How often should my son check his blood glucose levels?

Ideally, at least four times a day. Self-monitoring of blood glucose (SMBG) is an important part of daily diabetes care. In all kids with diabetes, pre-meal blood glucose numbers are used to figure out the overall diabetes treatment plan. Post-meal blood glucose values are helpful in determining the impact of food, especially carbohydrate, on blood glucose control. Checks before bed can help manage overnight glucose levels. Additionally, timed post-meal checks can measure the effectiveness of certain types of medications, such as rapid- or short-acting insulin, as well as certain oral medications that may be used for treating type 2 diabetes. Kids at risk for hypoglycemia (low blood glucose) should monitor their blood glucose levels whenever they suspect their glucose may be low. Teen drivers should perform a quick check to see whether or not blood glucose levels are in a safe range before getting behind the wheel. When the usual daily routine is altered, such as in the case of illness or changes in activity levels, blood glucose levels should be monitored closely to help with any necessary adjustments needed in your child's treatment plan.

Sixty Four

Is there a blood glucose meter that is considered "best" for my daughter to use?

Yes, the one that best suits her needs. There are several factors to consider when selecting a blood glucose monitor, which include:

- Accuracy
- Range of readings
- Time required to perform the check (may vary from 5 to 45 seconds)
- Ease of performing the test: how easy is it to apply the blood?
- Ease of use
- Cost of the strips and the meter
- Insurance coverage for the meter and supplies
- Availability of a memory function on the meter
- Test result download capabilities for the user and/or physician
- Manufacturer's warranty
- Available technical support

Taking the above factors into consideration can help you and your daughter select the meter that is right for her. Prior to purchasing a meter, discuss the options with her diabetes care team. They'll have experience with the meters available and can provide detailed training on the various types.

Sixty Five

My 9 year old hates doing finger-sticks. Are there other options?

Yes, but it still requires a "stick." Fingertips have traditionally been used for sampling blood glucose. However, several blood glucose meters on the market today offer "alternative-site testing." This method utilizes a lancet device that collects a blood sample from other sites, such as the forearm, thigh, or calf. The meters that work with alternative sampling sites are approved by the Food and Drug Administration (FDA) specifically for this use. Before purchasing one of these meters, find out which alternative sites can be used with that particular model. Not all meters are approved for the same sites and some sites may not be right for your child. These meters can usually be used with the fingertips in addition to the alternative site.

Be sure you and your child are instructed in proper use of the meter with the site that you are planning to use because the procedure and equipment may be different when sticking the alternative site as opposed to the fingertips. It is generally best to use the fingertips when a rapid change in blood glucose, such as hypoglycemia, occurs. Because blood flow to the finger or palm at the base of the thumb is generally three to five times faster than alternative sites, fingertip samples may show these changes sooner than other areas. Discuss with your child's diabetes care team whether alternative-site testing is an option for your child.

Sixty Six

What is the purpose of ketone testing?

To help evaluate your diabetes therapy. Ketosis is a condition of raised levels of ketones, which are a by-product of fat breakdown. When ketones are present, it indicates that the body is metabolizing fat for energy. This is not normal and can occur when blood glucose levels are very high. If not detected and remedied, this can lead to a dangerous condition called diabetic ketoacidosis (DKA).

Ketone monitoring can be done one of two ways. One option is by using urine monitoring strips that detect ketones in the urine. The other is by using a special test strip and meter that is designed for measuring blood ketones. Kids with diabetes should check for ketones during unexpected or persistent hyperglycemia, during illness, or during times of weight loss.

Ketones should be monitored whenever the blood glucose level is unexpectedly or repeatedly 240-300 mg/dl or higher. When a child is ill, the stress of the illness may cause the blood glucose levels to be quite higher than normal, which can increase the possibility of ketosis. Ketones should always be checked during any gastrointestinal illness regardless of the blood glucose result. Weight loss, whether intentional or unexpected, could be the result of hyperglycemia that needs to be corrected. When ketones are present during hyperglycemia, the condition must be promptly managed to avoid significant illness and possible hospitalization.

Sixty Seven

My 15-year-old daughter has been recording her own blood glucose values. When I look in the meter memory, there are no results for weeks. What should I do?

Ask her what happened and avoid accusing her of anything before your hear her answer. A question, such as "I noticed there are no glucose results in your meter memory for the last several weeks, will you tell me why?" gives her a chance to explain. It allows her to tell you why, and perhaps it will help you understand. She may have reasons that are perfectly valid to her, such as "they are always high" or "checking that often is too intense" or "my friends don't have to do it." Think about how you might feel if your blood glucose values were always high or if you had to check four times daily, often during times when your peers were around. Adolescents are struggling to find their own identity and, at this age, often face a period when diabetes management and blood glucose control become more difficult.

It does appear your daughter may not be monitoring her blood glucose levels, which can be the result of her efforts to distance herself and become more independent. Despite her struggle for independence, your daughter still needs your help. Slipping blood glucose control can have an impact on her future health. Let your daughter know that her health is important to you. Ask her diabetes care team to help you find ways to be supportive, yet involved. In the future, the diabetes care team may request that, when she comes in, she bring both her log book records and her meter with memory so that the data can be downloaded for comparison.

Sixty Eight

The pediatric endocrinologist recommended checking my son's blood glucose levels in the middle of the night. Is this really necessary?

It can be. Nocturnal or "middle of the night" blood glucose monitoring is generally recommended between 2:00 AM and 4:00 AM and these blood glucose values can provide very important clues to your son's treatment plan. These checks are often recommended when there is a big difference between bedtime and fasting (first thing in the morning) blood glucose levels. If that is the case, and the nocturnal check is higher than the bedtime reading, then your son's blood glucose may be rising in the middle of the night and contributing to the high morning blood glucose. In this case, an insulin adjustment, such as an increase in the basal regimen to help lower overnight blood glucose values, may be necessary. If the nocturnal check reveals the blood glucose level is too low, this hypoglycemia can be causing hormones in the body to be secreted and in turn causing the fasting blood glucose to be too high. This is referred to as "rebounding." If this happens, then the basal insulin regimen will likely need to be lowered to raise the middle-of-the-night value and hopefully avoid morning high blood glucose levels.

Anytime any adjustments are made to your son's basal insulin regimen, nocturnal monitoring may be recommended until the adjustment is satisfactory. Nocturnal monitoring may become more of a routine in kids with diabetes that have a tendency for hypoglycemia to occur in the middle of the night and/or in those who have hypoglycemia unawareness, meaning their body doesn't readily recognize the warning symptoms for hypoglycemia.

Sixty Nine

My 17 year old was just diagnosed with diabetes and blood glucose testing was recommended. I remember my mom checking her urine for glucose. Is this an option?

Not really. Monitoring glucose in the urine is no longer considered a useful way to monitor blood glucose levels for diabetes therapy. Monitoring glucose in the urine does just that; it only tells you whether or not glucose is present in the urine and doesn't give you an actual blood glucose value. Self-monitoring of blood glucose (SMBG), using blood samples and glucose meters, provides you and your son with actual blood glucose values, which can then be compared to blood glucose targets in an individual treatment plan. This method of blood glucose monitoring is much more accurate and much more useful in the management of diabetes.

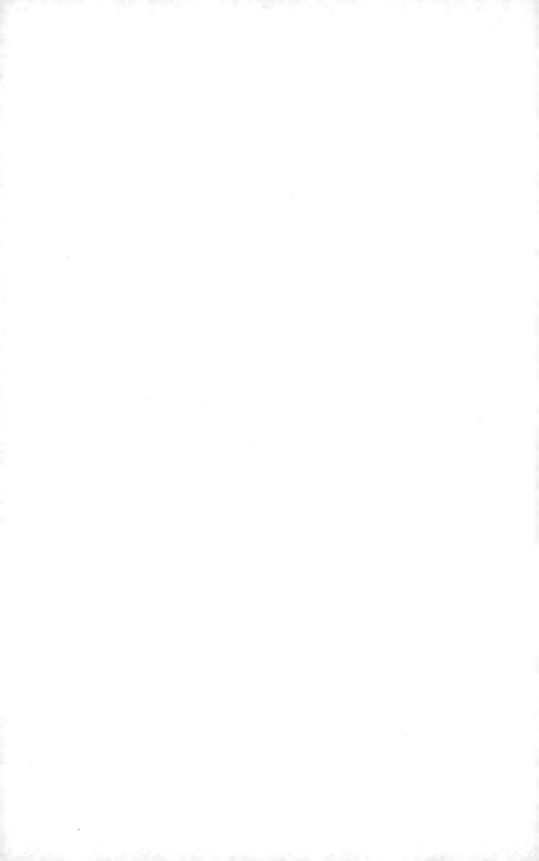

Chapter 10.
Psychosocial:
Living and Coping with Diabetes

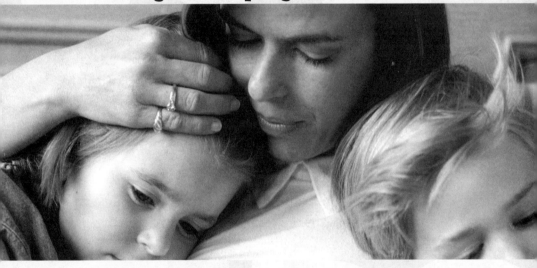

*T*he first few years after the diagnosis of diabetes tend to set the stage as to how diabetes will be handled by a child and his family. It is important to develop a strong support network, including a diabetes care team, to help determine the plan for dealing with diabetes in the most positive and productive manner.

Seventy

What are some ways to help my daughter with diabetes feel less "different" than other kids?

By helping her recognize that she is a kid first; she just also happens to have diabetes. Kids with diabetes may feel they are different from their peers and may be at risk for social difficulties. As a parent, you want her to maintain a positive social environment while staying healthy. Following are some guidelines for helping your daughter feel less at odds with her peers:

- Keep her involved in social activities, especially with others her age.
- Identify any challenges in the social environment.
- Attend school regularly.
- Participate in school activities.
- Allow her to play sports, if she desires.
- Develop a plan for managing diabetes in the school setting.
- Acknowledge peer pressure can interfere with diabetes tasks.
- Recognize conflicts that result from peer pressure.
- If needed, seek help from a counselor.

Keep in mind that she will still need help with diabetes management during the course of normal kid activities. Continue to rely on her diabetes care team, an excellent resource for this type of experience and expertise.

Seventy One

My husband and I are divorced. How should we deal with our son's diagnosis of diabetes?

By focusing on his best interests. The following ideas may help you stay unified with regards to your son's diabetes care needs:

- Recognize education and training for your son's diabetes treatment plan is an important and ongoing process for all of you.
- Plan on one parent from each family attending diabetes care team visits with him.
- Communicate frequently. Keep your child involved in his diabetes care in both households and don't rely on him to be the only one to relay information back and forth.
- Keep diabetes supplies in both homes; things such as insulin and necessary medications; insulin syringes and/or insulin pump infusion sets; blood glucose monitoring and ketone testing supplies; glucose tablets and, if necessary, a glucagon emergency kit; and any other appropriate items.
- If your child attends school, both of you should become familiar with the plan for dealing with his diabetes in this setting, making sure the school has all necessary contact information for both families.
- Deal with any conflict between you and your ex-husband outside your son's environment.

Your child needs established family support. All of you can draw on this strength to successfully manage the challenges of diabetes.

Seventy Two

My daughter has type 2 diabetes and is being teased about her weight. What should I do?

Tell her to walk away. No child deserves to be teased about anything, especially when it makes them uncomfortable. Developing a positive support system is important. It may be helpful for your daughter to meet other kids with diabetes that have some of the same concerns that she has. Some suggestions may include:

- Find a support group. Many hospitals, health-focused centers, or outpatient clinics have programs for kids with both types of diabetes.
- Check out the nearest diabetes camp (see page 109). Your daughter will meet other kids with diabetes, perhaps her own age and with the same type of diabetes.
- If she wants to lose weight, find a resource that is right for her. A dietitian that works with kids that want to lose weight may offer additional education and support.
- Encourage her to learn all she can about diabetes. Magazines, such as *Diabetes Forecast*®, have resources for kids with diabetes and may offer solutions for healthy eating.

Dealing with a chronic illness, as well as being teased about weight, can create pressure for any kid dealing with diabetes. Reach out for help, if needed. Her diabetes care team may recommend a counselor to help her develop healthy coping strategies and stay focused with a positive self-esteem.

Seventy Three

My 15-year-old daughter has type 1 diabetes and is obsessed with her weight. I've noticed her blood glucose is constantly high. What can I do?

Seek professional advice immediately. Body image is very important to adolescents. If your daughter is "obsessed" or unhappy with her weight, she may resort to lowering or not taking her insulin dose so her blood glucose levels remain constantly high. This results in a loss of glucose and calories through the urine, which leads to weight loss. Other behaviors related to eating disorders include severely limiting food and an extreme fixation on exercise. Regardless of how it shows up, if an eating disorder is present, it needs to be addressed right away. Start with her diabetes care team. The team will assess your daughter's behavior and evaluate the effectiveness of her overall diabetes treatment plan. Counseling or psychotherapy may help identify stress factors that lead your daughter to lose weight at the risk of her health. Most importantly, focus on healthy strategies that achieve a proper weight and good blood glucose control.

Seventy Four

Several of our relatives are constantly telling my son that they "feel sorry for him" because he has diabetes. Is there anything I can or should do?

Ask them to stop. Tell them that your son's focus is living healthy with diabetes and that "feeling sorry for him" does not help. These feelings may seem natural to them and they may not realize they're having a negative impact on your son. Suggest that they educate themselves about diabetes (*www.diabetes.org*). Relatives that are around your son more often may benefit from learning specific information about his treatment plan. Increasing their knowledge may not only help them to better understand it, but also increase their awareness of the bright future your son has by staying healthy with diabetes. If relatives continue to "feel sorry for him" after the request to stop and the education efforts, then you may have to distance your son from them to avoid such comments.

Seventy Five

My child's endocrinologist recommended a psychologist see her. Is something wrong?

Not necessarily. A mental health professional, such as a psychologist, behaviorist, or social worker, is considered part of the diabetes care team. Chronic conditions that require constant self-care, such as diabetes, can have a huge emotional impact on a person and his or her family. Research has shown the benefit of a mental health professional in the care of those with a chronic illness. The endocrinologist is likely recommending this resource to help your son focus on the positives in his environment, as well as identify the presence of any characteristics that may affect your son's diabetes negatively. Negative influences on a child's diabetes can be the presence of another illness, such as asthma; issues such as eating disorders; and emotional and behavioral problems such as delinquent behavior and even depression. If a child doesn't have enough parental support, has a family history of depression or mental disorders, or lacks health insurance, all of these factors can negatively influence diabetes care. In some cases, life events that affect parents, such as job changes or death in the family, can disrupt diabetes management in children. The psychologist can help your child and family deal with diabetes in a way that contributes to a healthy environment for your child with diabetes.

Chapter 11.
School Days:
Factoring Diabetes into the Equation

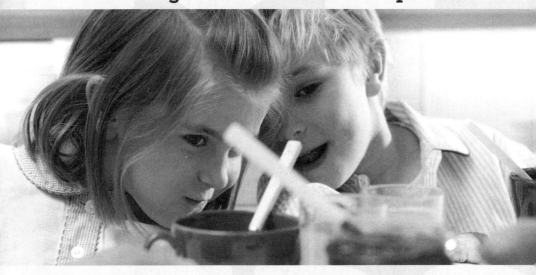

*S*chool can present significant challenges or be a source of support for kids with diabetes. Planning for safety and health is the key to making school a supportive environment. It is important to encourage kids to attend school regularly and to participate in school activities and sports to facilitate as normal an academic and social environment as possible.

Seventy Six

My child's endocrinologist mentioned a "504 plan." Why is this important?

It preserves your child's rights in the school setting. Kids with diabetes are protected by federal law, and a formal plan called a "504 plan," which refers to section 504 of the Rehabilitation Act of 1973, can outline your child's specific diabetes care needs during school hours. Your own plan for diabetes care should outline:

- Who is trained and will supervise care in the school setting
- Location of necessary diabetes supplies
- Schedule and location for blood glucose monitoring and medication administration
- Signs, symptoms, and treatment for hypoglycemia
- Signs, symptoms, and treatment for hyperglycemia
- Timing of meals and snacks
- The need for free access to the restroom and water fountain
- Accommodations for changes in routine and physical activity
- Permission for excused absences for diabetes medical care
- Emergency contact information and what to do in emergencies

The 504 plan may be requested by the school, by the parent or guardian, or in a situation where there is a problem with the child's diabetes care in the school setting. Ideally, the plan is developed ahead of time. You can find a sample of the section 504 plan on the American Diabetes Association's website at *www.diabetes.org*.

Seventy
Seven

Should my son with diabetes eat lunch in the school cafeteria?

If he prefers. Since your son has diabetes, you're probably concerned that he's eating healthy and maintaining blood glucose targets. The school cafeteria can make this easier. Menus for both breakfast and lunch meals provided by the school cafeteria are often pre-set and available ahead of time. You and your son can use the menus to figure out the amount of carbohydrate in the foods that are offered in the school menu and see how the meal might fit into his diabetes treatment plan. This can also be an opportunity for your son to learn about healthy food choices.

The Food Service Manager at the school should be included in any training regarding your son's diabetes care plan. Training should include his type of diabetes meal plan; signs, symptoms, and treatment of hypoglycemia; and the importance of timing meals and providing enough time to finish his meal. The Food Service Manager should also be able to provide the nutrition information that is available for meals served and keep you informed about any changes in school lunch menus.

Seventy Eight

My daughter wants to ride home on the school bus. What if something happens related to her diabetes?

Hopefully, with proper planning, any diabetes-related events can be minimal. With that said, if your daughter is going to be riding the school bus, then it is important to include her school bus driver in any necessary training regarding her diabetes care plan. Getting to know the school bus driver, as well as any other drivers that may drive the route, is a good idea. Make sure the bus driver:

- Knows your child by name and knows that she has diabetes
- Knows the schedule for when your daughter rides the bus
- Has a copy of her emergency contact information/plan on the bus in a secure place and available to alternate drivers
- Knows the signs, symptoms, and treatment for hypoglycemia
- Knows the signs, symptoms, and treatment for hyperglycemia
- Has supplies for treatment of hypoglycemia in a designated location on the bus
- Is familiar with where your daughter keeps her diabetes supplies when riding the bus
- Allows your daughter snacks while riding the bus
- Reports any diabetes-related events to school personnel and/or family members
- Treats the student as other children riding the school bus, while responding to diabetes needs when necessary
- Respects her privacy and confidentiality

Seventy
Nine

Recently, my daughter had a health screening by the school nurse and has "acanthosis nigricans." What does that mean?

Acanthosis nigricans is a sign of insulin resistance. It is character-ized by darkening of the skin in the folds of the neck, armpits, or groin and in many cases is accompanied by obesity. It is associated with hyperinsulinemia, or insulin levels that are higher than normal in the bloodstream. Acanthosis nigricans is common in those with pre-diabetes or type 2 diabetes. It is more common in certain ethnic groups, particularly Native Americans, African Americans, and Hispanic Americans. The appearance of acanthosis nigricans can usu-ally be improved by adopting lifestyle changes that include healthy eating, increased physical activity, and weight loss. Healthy lifestyle changes also delay the onset of type 2 diabetes in those at risk, or if diabetes is present, can help improve blood glucose control.

Eighty

I have heard that diabetes affects concentration. Will my son's grades take a turn for the worse?

Diabetes-related events such as hypoglycemia and hyperglycemia can affect concentration. When blood glucose levels are too low, and a lack of glucose is available to the brain, symptoms such as trouble concentrating, changes in vision, slurred speech, lack of coordination, headaches, dizziness, and drowsiness will eventually occur. By treating hypoglycemia when milder symptoms (weakness, shakiness, clamminess, and increased heart rate) first show up, your son can avoid depriving his brain of glucose. Also, if your son has trouble recognizing hypoglycemia, more frequent blood glucose checks may help identify and promptly treat any hypoglycemia.

Hyperglycemia can also have an effect on your son's classroom situation. Symptoms of high blood glucose include blurred vision and fatigue, which can affect concentration. High glucose symptoms, such as dry mouth and frequent urination, can also cause your son to take extra trips to the water fountain and restroom, which disrupt classroom activity. When blood glucose levels are high a lot or when the level is extremely high, the consequences can be very serious and include vomiting, deep breathing, or loss of consciousness.

If hypoglycemia or hyperglycemia is common, you should immediately get in touch with his diabetes care team to determine what's causing this and the need for any changes in his treatment plan. Keeping his blood glucose levels in the best possible control and avoiding any diabetes-related interference can help keep his concentration (and hopefully his grades) top-notch while at school.

Eighty One

My first grader has physical education class mid-morning. What can we do to prevent the low blood glucose levels that occur soon after?

It depends. Exercise accounts for 10-20% of hypoglycemic episodes in children and adolescents. Often, these lows occur as the result of an increase in the usual intensity, duration, or frequency of activity. For children that exercise on a regular basis, adjusting diabetes medications, if necessary, is the preferred method for preventing hypoglycemia. Eating extra calories is also an option, but can be a problem when weight control is an issue. Your child's diabetes care team may recommend that his blood glucose be checked both before and after exercise to determine if any changes need to be made. If blood glucose levels are less than 100 mg/dl during periods of exercise, your child should eat 15 grams of carbohydrate.

Include your child's physical education teacher in any training regarding your child's individual diabetes care plan. Discuss the usual symptoms of hypoglycemia, the need for prompt blood glucose testing when necessary, and the need for access to carbohydrate for treatment of any hypoglycemic episodes. Children with diabetes who take insulin should also have a glucagon emergency kit (see page 60) available for treatment of severe hypoglycemia, should it occur.

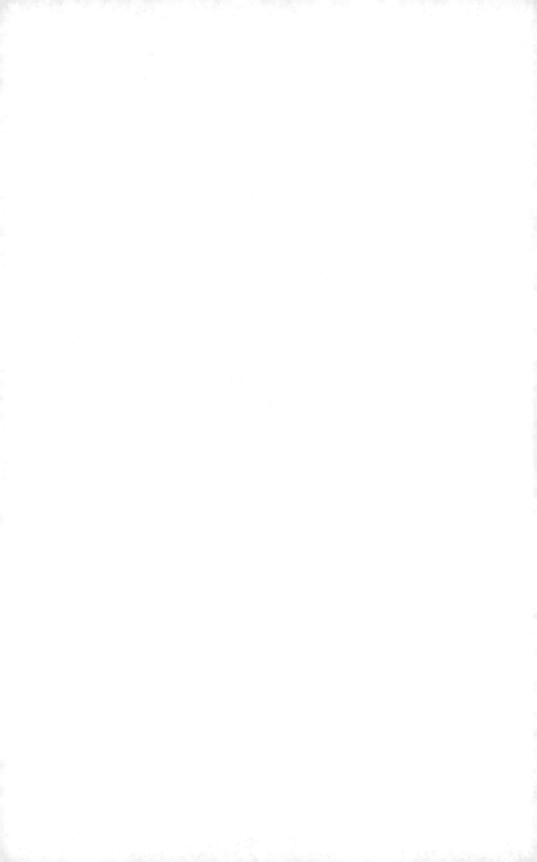

Chapter 12.
Athletes with Diabetes:
Champions and Challenges

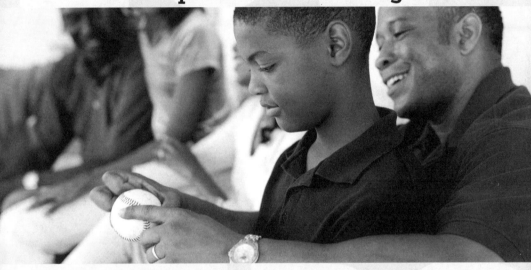

*D*iabetes should not be a barrier to participation in organized sports—it's just another factor to consider, much like appropriate footwear and pre-game meals. With the proper preparation and care, your child can achieve athletic goals at the highest level.

Eighty Two

Do various sports affect diabetes differently?

Yes. All physical activity lowers blood glucose, but various factors influence the way in which a specific sport affects diabetes. No matter what sport, always check blood glucose before, during, and after exercise.

Endurance sports (running, jogging, soccer, swimming) generally use carbohydrate as fuel when intense and more body fat when casual. It's especially important to have enough carbohydrate and less insulin to prevent hypoglycemia. In general, 15-30 grams of carbohydrate for every 30-60 minutes of activity is needed. More intense activities done in a shorter time frame may not require as much carbohydrate.

Power sports (basketball, baseball/softball, football, gymnastics, wrestling) require short, powerful bursts of activity that may only have a small effect on blood glucose. The position your child plays has a great deal to do with his requirements. Also be aware of the differing intensity levels between brief games and prolonged practices.

Fitness activities (aerobics, stationary bike, yoga, martial arts) vary widely in their intensity. Over time, as your son develops muscle mass and becomes more fit, his insulin sensitivity will improve, leading to lower insulin requirements.

Recreational sports (horseback riding, skiing, golf, tennis) can require reduced insulin doses and extra carbohydrate if they are intense (playing a singles tennis match) or can require no changes at all if they are steady, low-intensity activities such as golf.

Eighty Three

My son wants to try out for football. Is it safe for him to play?

Yes, with a little extra care. Athletes with diabetes are active at all levels of football, from recreational to professional. He can safely play football if you keep a few factors in mind:

- Football is a "power sport," which requires short, intense bursts of energy. Your son's blood glucose response and the need to adjust his food and medication will depend on which position he plays. Positions that require more running (wide receiver, defensive back) may cause a lower drop in blood glucose during a game than strength positions (offensive and defensive linemen). In either case, consider reducing insulin during practice/game time and for a few hours following. Have your son check his blood glucose before a game or practice and eat a small snack if it's less than 150 mg/dl. He should eat carbohydrate immediately after a strenuous workout or game to refill his glycogen stores.

- Practice may differ quite a bit from games in the amount of energy expended and blood glucose response. Because practices tend to be more intense and longer than games—particularly preseason "two a day" practices—your son may need to make more adjustments in food and medication.

- Your son will have the same risk for football-related injuries as other players, but he may have a longer recovery period or more infections related to his injuries unless his blood glucose is kept as near normal as possible.

Eighty Four

My daughter is an all-star softball player and wants an insulin pump. Could she wear it during her games?

Wearing an insulin pump during a game is an individual decision and depends on the participation policy of her league. If your daughter chooses to wear her pump, she should set her insulin infusion rate about 10-15% lower during the game and for 4-6 hours afterward to decrease her risk for hypoglycemia. She could also choose to use the "suspend" mode on her pump or even disconnect it and take a small injection or bolus of insulin (usually about half the normal amount) before a softball game, letting the physical activity control her blood glucose levels. Whatever approach she chooses should be based on careful blood glucose monitoring and a discussion with her diabetes care team.

Softball is a power sport in which your daughter may be sedentary for much of the game, but then experience short bursts of movement such as sprinting, hitting, and throwing. If she is a pitcher or catcher, she will be more active during a game than a player in the outfield. Practices may be more active than games, especially if there are a lot of running and conditioning drills. This activity may lead to hypoglycemia. Frequent blood glucose checks with adjustments in food and medication are important, no matter what your daughter decides about using an insulin pump to control her diabetes.

Eighty Five

Our recently diagnosed son has always been active in sports. Are there any famous athletes with diabetes? Where can we find information on sports and diabetes?

Athletes with both types of diabetes excel in every sport. A few of the better-known athletes with diabetes include:

Jason Johnson (baseball)

Scott Verplank (golf)

Adam Morrison (basketball)

Will Cross (extreme adventurer)

Chris Dudley (basketball)

Mike Echols (football)

Kris Freeman (cross-country skiing)

Gary Hall (swimming)

Kelli Kuehne (golf)

Jay Leeuwenburg (football)

Shannon Standridge (triathlete)

Dave Weingard (triathlete)

For more information on athletics and diabetes, try *The Diabetic Athlete* by Sheri Colberg, PhD. In addition, the Diabetes Exercise & Sports Association (DESA) has been a source of reliable information on physical fitness, exercise, and sports for people with diabetes for over 20 years. Their website (*www.diabetes-exercise.org*) is aimed at sports-minded individuals with diabetes and promotes networking, support, and sharing of information on healthy and safe exercise.

Eighty Six

We know an intense soccer game can cause my daughter's blood glucose to drop. What precautions should we take and what should we tell her coach and teammates?

There are a variety of things to do. Your daughter should check her blood glucose before the game and if it's less than 150 mg/dl, she should eat a small snack. Generally, 15–30 grams of carbohydrate is needed for each 30-60 minutes of physical activity. Also, check blood glucose periodically throughout the game and immediately if symptoms of hypoglycemia occur. Fifteen grams of readily absorbed sugar, such as a sports drink or fresh fruit, should be given if at any time her blood glucose drops lower than 100 mg/dl. You may also want to consider lowering her insulin dose; if your daughter is on an insulin pump, it may be necessary to lower her basal rate for 4-6 hours after the game to prevent post-exercise hypoglycemia.

Your daughter should wear some form of medical alert identification that indicates she has diabetes. Her soccer coach and perhaps a teammate or two also need to know that she has diabetes, as well as a few basic facts about blood glucose checks; symptoms and treatment of hypoglycemia; and the need for extra food.

As a parent, you are responsible for your daughter having her blood glucose monitoring equipment, glucose tablets, hard candy or juice, water, and snacks close by during the game. Encourage your child to wear medical identification and to stop exercising and check her blood glucose at the earliest sign of hypoglycemia. Taking a few precautions will help your daughter play soccer safely and have fun doing it!

Chapter 13.
Special Events:
No Kid-ding Around

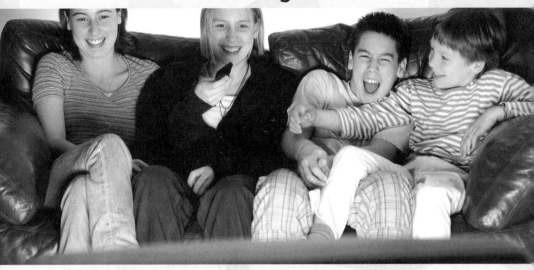

*A*s kids grow up, they become more confident and increasingly social. The respect of their peer group becomes more important to their self-esteem as well as the development of their personal sense of identity.

Eighty Seven

At what age should I allow my daughter with diabetes to spend the night with friends?

Whenever both you and she are ready. It is important that your daughter feel comfortable enough with her diabetes skills that she, along with some supervision from an adult in that setting, can manage the sleepover situation. In addition, you need to feel comfortable in letting her go. Preparation can be the key to safety and success. Consider the following when planning this event:

- How much do the adults (parents) in charge of the sleepover know about diabetes?
- What can you do to educate them about your daughter's diabetes plan?
- Develop a "diabetes care kit" that keeps all her diabetes supplies (with any instructions needed) in one location.
- Work with your daughter to role-play any situations that could occur (such as hypoglycemia or non-planned snacks).
- Have your contact information available at the house where the sleepover is located.

Talk to your daughter's diabetes care team for advice. Ask them for suggestions to make sure your daughter's overnight stay is safe and comfortable for all parties involved.

Eighty Eight

My son wants to go to diabetes camp. Is this a good idea?

Yes. Diabetes camp is an opportunity for your son to meet other kids that have diabetes. Your son would be in a medically supervised environment, while enjoying the fun that camp itself can provide. Similar to most camps, diabetes camp offers the usual activities while at the same time providing coaching and education on personal diabetes self-management skills. Many kids that attend diabetes camp go on to be camp counselors, which is a great opportunity to become a mentor to younger kids with diabetes.

The American Diabetes Association and its camping partners are the largest providers of camps for children with diabetes in the world. If you are interested in detailed information about diabetes camp, you may want to read the American Diabetes Association's *Getting the Most Out of Diabetes Camp*. This book provides tips for selecting the right camp, ways to determine if your child is ready for camp, and step-by-step help with the application process. Also, it includes a sample application packet, packing lists, and more.

Eighty Nine

The snacks and treats at holiday parties are a challenge for my son with diabetes. Any suggestions?

The key is to have fun and enjoy the party without sacrificing his glucose control. You may want to talk with the host of the party ahead of time to see what snacks and treats will be available. This way you can choose what might work best with your son's diabetes treatment plan. In addition, you could offer to bring one or two snacks that are tasty—as well as healthy—for your son and his friends to enjoy. It may also be helpful to verify what types of activities are planned for the party. If your son will be more active than usual, such as with skating or rock-climbing, a little extra carbohydrate might be okay and fit within his treatment plan. If the party is more of a sit-down type of get-together and focused on eating, then you may want to adjust your son's medication to fit in something like a small piece of birthday cake. Rather than say no to any item of food, you and your son can plan for and balance his treatment plan to best meet his needs that day.

Ninety

It seems that at most social events my teen attends pizza is the food of choice. How can we manage the havoc it wreaks on her blood glucose control?

Carefully. Pizza is an interesting case and there has actually been research done to examine the effect of pizza on blood glucose levels. In the study, on two separate evenings, subjects ate meals that were similar in carbohydrate, fat, and protein. One meal was pizza and the other was a "control" meal that included other foods that had similar nutrients to pizza. The same amount of insulin was taken for both meals. The results showed that, directly after eating, glucose was reasonably controlled with both meals. However, blood glucose levels continued to rise and were much higher anywhere from 4 to 9 hours after the pizza, as compared to the control meal. The researchers concluded that perhaps pizza has properties that cause an increase in after-meal (post-pizza) blood glucose for as much as 9 hours later. Knowing this, your daughter will need to monitor her blood glucose levels for several hours after she eats pizza and track the changes that occur. This will help your daughter and her diabetes team develop a plan to minimize the "havoc," perhaps with additional exercise, changes in her medication regimen, and/or changing the amount of pizza she eats to keep her blood glucose control in the target range.

Ninety
One

We're planning our first family vacation since my daughter was diagnosed with diabetes. Any helpful suggestions?

Plan for your daughter's health as much as you plan for your trip. Checking blood glucose every few hours during the trip, especially on travel days, helps monitor any changes in control. When packing, keep the following items in mind:

- Medical Alert Tag
- Medications, as well as any insulin syringes or infusion sets needed (at least double the amount necessary) with prescription labeling to confirm the medical necessity of these items
- Diabetes management supplies (meter, extra batteries, test strips, lancet device, lancets, urine ketone strips if your daughter has type 1 diabetes) in ample amounts
- Treatment for hypoglycemia (if needed), such as glucose tablets or hard candy
- Glucagon emergency kit (if recommended by your doctor)
- Important phone numbers, including your pharmacy's
- Medical insurance card and/or information for travel insurance
- List of local medical facilities and resources at your destination
- Snacks that are stable in the travel environment
- Comfortable shoes   .

Also be sure that all family members know the location of your daughter's diabetes supplies

Ninety Two

Since she was diagnosed with diabetes, I'm afraid to let my child go trick-or-treating on Halloween. Is this reasonable or am I being silly?

This isn't silly, you're just being a concerned parent. You're probably scared the temptation of Halloween treats could upset your daughter's blood glucose control. If your daughter wants, there's no reason why she should not participate in Halloween fun. Some suggestions to help you plan a safe and happy Halloween:

- Focus on the costume and not the candy. Plan activities around the experience of "dressing up" for Halloween.
- Plan a party. You and your daughter can plan the menu with tasty snacks that best fit into her diabetes treatment plan.
- Activities like going to a haunted house or a hayride can add to the Halloween spirit.
- Kids with diabetes should be able to trick-or-treat if they enjoy it. Just keep in mind that not only is most candy filled with sugar, it's usually filled with empty calories as well.
- Perhaps your daughter can pick a few favorite treats and then share the others with an orphanage or nursing home (individually wrapped and with permission, of course).
- Treats other than candy are nice. Stickers, word puzzles, and small toys are a few ideas that are popular with kids.

Ask your daughter's diabetes care team for advice on planning for events such as Halloween. With a little bit of planning, your daughter can enjoy a safe and happy Halloween.

Chapter 14.
Ongoing Care:
Successful Diabetes Self-Management

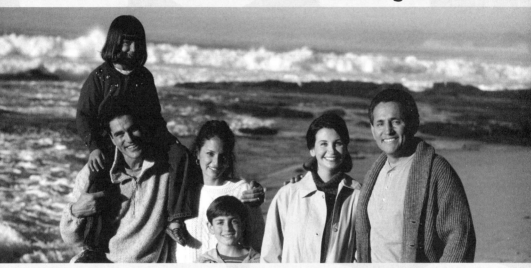

Successful diabetes care is essentially self-care. While the medical team develops the treatment plan, the child with diabetes and his or her family is responsible for the daily implementation of that plan. Learning to handle the day-to-day challenges of life with diabetes is key to successful diabetes self-management.

Ninety Three

When should I give my child more responsibility for taking care of his diabetes?

Whenever you feel your child is ready. Successful diabetes self-management is a healthy balance between your responsibilities as a parent and those of your child. There is no standard recommended age at which a child is capable of assuming more responsibility for his diabetes care; the transition varies based on motor development, reasoning abilities, and emotional maturity.

Of course, the parents of infants and toddlers with diabetes assume all of the responsibilities of diabetes management for their child. While preschoolers may lack most of the skills to take charge of self-care, they can still help with blood glucose checks, record keeping, and tracking carbohydrate intake. School-aged children still need a lot of supervision, but can begin to help with insulin injections and blood glucose monitoring. Adolescents are capable of performing self-management tasks, but still need help with decision-making, especially with insulin adjustment and managing sick days.

Parents should look for opportunities to teach skills, such as blood glucose monitoring, carbohydrate counting, and insulin injections, followed by a chance for the child to demonstrate his ability. The goal of diabetes self-management in children is a partnership between parent and child, with a gradual transition to independent management by your child.

Ninety
Four

My child has had diabetes for 3 years. When should she see an ophthalmologist? How often should we have her kidneys checked?

The American Diabetes Association has developed Standards of Care, describing the basic care a person with diabetes needs.

At diagnosis:
• Establish goals of care and treatment
• Begin diabetes self-management education
• Provide nutritional therapy by a registered dietitian
• Conduct a psychosocial assessment

At each quarterly visit, check:
• A1C
• Growth (height and weight) and body mass index (BMI)
• Blood pressure
• Self-monitoring blood glucose records
• Psychosocial assessment
• Injection sites

Once a year, have:
• Nutrition therapy evaluation
• Microalbuminuria test–if 10 years old and has had diabetes for 5 years
• Ophthalmologic examination–if 10 years or older and has had diabetes for 3-5 years, then repeated annually
• Thyroid function test–at diagnosis and every 1-2 years thereafter
• Depression screening–for children 10 years of age or older
• Complete foot evaluation
• Influenza vaccination
• Lipid check

Ninety Five

How should we handle sick days? Should we still give our son his insulin, even if he isn't eating well?

Children with diabetes need special care when they are ill. Sick-day issues include avoiding hyperglycemia and hypoglycemia, and preventing diabetic ketoacidosis (DKA). Monitor blood glucose every few hours, check ketones frequently, and make sure your child gets plenty of fluid. If ketones are present, call your health care team for advice. Ketones are an indication that the body does not have enough insulin, and this lack of insulin can lead to DKA, a serious situation that can cause coma and death if left untreated.

It is difficult to predict the effect of illness on insulin needs. A poor appetite or nausea and vomiting may lead to less food and less insulin needs. But, an older child's glucose levels rise due to the release of stress hormones and glycogen, a form of stored glucose. Infants and young children don't have the ability to store and release much glycogen, so their blood glucose may run low.

Food on sick days needs to be as close to the meal plan as possible, although an upset stomach may require substitutions. Try to keep mealtime and carbohydrate content at each feeding similar to a normal day. Use liquids that contain carbohydrate in the appropriate amounts, such as sports drinks, juices, gelatin, broth, and popsicles.

The best preparation for sick days takes place in advance. Establish a sick-day plan that includes directions for reaching the physician, guidance on administering insulin or oral medication, recommendations for blood and urine testing, and suggested foods for sick days.

Ninety Six

How can we tell if our daughter's blood glucose is low? What should we do to raise it to a safe level?

Signs of low blood glucose include hunger, nervousness and shakiness, sweating, light-headedness, sleepiness, confusion, and anxiety. Hypoglycemia may be difficult to recognize or confused with bad behavior in a young child. Causes of hypoglycemia include less carbohydrate than usual in a meal or snack, missing a meal or snack, extra activity, too much insulin, side effects of other medications, or drinking alcoholic beverages, especially on an empty stomach. This lack of glucose can affect the brain and nerve cells, particularly if blood glucose levels are below 60 mg/dl. If left untreated, unconsciousness or a seizure can develop. Guidelines for treatment are based on severity.

Mild hypoglycemia, with symptoms such as sweating, pallor, tremors, headache, and behavior change, can be treated by the child by eating 15 grams of easily absorbed carbohydrate (3–4 glucose tablets, 1/2 cup fruit juice or regular soft drink, 2 teaspoons of sugar or honey) followed by a snack. Check glucose again 15 minutes after treatment.

Moderate hypoglycemia, with symptoms such as aggressiveness, drowsiness, and confusion, requires treatment be given by someone other than the child, but the treatment can usually be given orally.

Severe hypoglycemia is associated with coma, seizures, and the inability to take glucose orally. In this case, your child may need a shot of glucagon (see page 60) or intravenous glucose administered by a health care professional.

Ninety Seven

How can we tell if our daughter's blood glucose is high? Is this an emergency?

The symptoms of hyperglycemia (high blood glucose) are frequent urination, excess hunger and thirst, and fatigue. If blood glucose is high, the body may begin producing ketones, which appear when the body burns fat instead of glucose. Excess ketones in the blood and urine can lead to diabetic ketoacidosis (DKA), a serious situation in which the blood can turn acidic and cause coma and death if left untreated.

Hyperglycemia can be caused by eating more carbohydrate than usual in a meal or snack, inactivity, not enough diabetes medication, side effects of other medication, infection or illness such as a cold or flu, as well as stress and changes in hormone levels, such as during menstrual periods.

Occasional high blood glucose levels are to be expected, but if high blood glucose continues on a chronic basis, poor growth, persistent infections, and complications of diabetes can occur. Checking blood glucose levels often and attempting to keep them within the target range will enable you to become aware of hyperglycemia early and adjust your child's medication dose, food intake, or physical activity as needed.

Ninety
Eight

Should our son with diabetes wear a medical identification tag?

Yes. Everyone who has diabetes should always wear a medical identification tag. The information on the tag could save your son's life in an emergency.

Medic alert bracelets and necklaces are available in pharmacies or from other organizations; fashionable alternatives can also be found on the Internet. Infants and young children should not wear identification necklaces as they may pose a hazard. Shoe ID tags may be useful for toddlers. Wallet ID cards are not necessarily a good substitute, since these can easily be missed by emergency personnel. It is especially important that teenagers who are driving and are often away from home wear medical identification, as should children who are active in sports.

Ninety Nine

Should our child with diabetes take a flu shot every year?

Yes, because people with diabetes have an increased risk for hospitalization due to influenza and its complications. Although flu shots will not give your child 100% protection from the flu, the vaccination should be given to children with diabetes who are over 6 months of age. The best time to get the flu shot is in the early fall, since it needs about 2 weeks to take effect.

A pneumonia shot is also recommended for children with diabetes age 2 or older. The pneumonia shot can also protect from other infections such as meningitis or bacteremia. The pneumonia shot can be given any time during the year and, for most people, one shot is enough protection for a lifetime.

One Hundred

We're concerned our son may engage in some risky behaviors, such as drinking, smoking, and drug use. How can these behaviors affect his diabetes control?

All of these behaviors are unhealthy in general, but they pose special risks for your teen with diabetes. Remember that teenagers with diabetes have the same drive for independence as other teenagers and may also face the temptation to ignore their diabetes care and act like everyone else.

Alcohol is a special risk for people with diabetes for a number of reasons. Drinking alcohol, particularly without eating, causes hypoglycemia. Symptoms of hypoglycemia can also resemble alcohol intoxication, perhaps leading to delayed treatment. A teenager with diabetes who has been drinking may also forget his care plan or neglect to treat hypoglycemia.

Smoking is linked to lung cancer as well as heart disease, and people with diabetes already have a higher than average risk of getting heart disease, high blood pressure, and kidney disease. Combining smoking with diabetes compounds these risks.

Illegal drugs can alter blood glucose levels, lowering them in some cases and raising them in others. Marijuana use can increase hunger, leading to overeating and high blood glucose levels. It's also linked to indifference, which can cause your son to ignore his care plan.

If you think your teenager is engaged in risky behaviors, keep the lines of communication open and try to be as patient as possible. Certainly you should make your teenager aware of the potential poor effects of risky behaviors on his diabetes control, yet be aware of his activities and remain supportive of his need for independence.

One Hundred One

Recently, our teenage daughter has become uncomfortable going to the pediatrician. How can we help her make a good transition to an adult health care setting?

The transition to adult care providers should be planned and negotiated among your daughter, your family, the pediatric diabetes team, and the adult care providers. While some teenagers with diabetes remain comfortable with their pediatric diabetes teams for quite some time, others are ready to move into a more adult setting at an earlier age.

By the time your daughter is 16 years old, you need to start discussing this transition with her and her current health care team. Involve your teenage daughter from the beginning in the search for a new caregiver and ask your current team to suggest health care professionals for you and your daughter to consider. Help her make an appointment for a pre-transfer visit, and use this visit to evaluate the features of the clinic, treatment practices, and personalities of the health care team she'll be using before making a final decision. After she makes her decision, it is helpful if her pediatrician writes a formal letter of referral to her new physician, summarizing her history and current care plan in addition to transferring her medical records.

INDEX

A1C scores, 39, 74-76

Acanthosis nigricans, 97

ACE-inhibitors, 64

Adolescents with diabetes, 6, 35-41, 81
  risky behaviors by, 123
  transitioning from pediatric to adult, 124

Alcohol use, 123

American Diabetes Association (ADA)
  recommended testing protocol, 117
  website of, 9, 18, 90, 94

Athletes with diabetes, 6, 101-106
  types of sports, 102-103

Babies with diabetes, 13-19
  checking blood glucose levels in, 15
  irritability in, 14

Basal insulin doses, 45, 57, 82

Blood glucose levels, 2-3
  controlling, 5, 38, 81, 89
  safe target range for, 16, 69, 74-75, 111

Blood glucose monitoring, 2-3, 6, 14, 25, 73-83
  with exercise, 68-71
  frequency of, 77, 102-104, 106
  meters for, 78
  nocturnal, 82

Body image, 89

Bolus insulin doses, 45, 49, 57

Books recommended, vii, 8, 22, 49, 105, 109

Calories, 48

Camping and hiking, 112

Carbohydrates, 44, 48, 70-72

Children with diabetes
  being teased in school, 31, 53, 88

developing independence in, 24-26, 81
  giving choices to, 19, 59
  involving in their own care, 21, 33, 116
  "job description," 22
  praising, 8, 19, 23
  rewarding, 7, 23
  risky behaviors by, 123
  supervising and supporting, 33, 85-91
  teaching about diabetes, 25, 38, 116

Correction bolus, 57

Counseling assistance, 10, 31, 86, 91

Depression, professional help for, 10, 91

Diabetes
  ADA Standards of Care, 117
  affect on ability to concentrate, 98
  individualizing care for, 1-11
  no "cure" for, 4

Diabetes camps, 31, 88, 109

"Diabetes care kit," developing, 108

Diabetes Control and Complications Trial
  (DCCT), 4-5

Diabetes education, vii, 9, 63
  for caregivers, coaches, teachers, and
    friends, 18, 24, 60, 106
  for the child, 25, 38, 79, 116
  for insensitive relatives, 90
  for the physical education teacher, 99
  for the school bus driver, 96

Diabetes Exercise & Sports Association
  (DESA), 105

Diabetes self-management, 115-124

Diabetic ketoacidosis, 69, 80

Drug use (illegal), 123

Eating disorders, 36, 89, 91

Eating healthy foods, 3-4, 25, 43-53. *See also* Portion size

    at parties, 110

    in restaurants, 49

    in the school cafeteria, 95

Environmental triggers, 2, 11

Ethnicity. *See* individual racial and ethnic groups

Exercise. *See* Physical activity and exercise

Family history. *See* Genetic causes

Family support, 66, 87, 91

Fat (dietary), 46

Fears, 10

Fiber (dietary), 48

"504" plans, 94

Flu shots, 122

Food pyramid, 51

Football, and diabetes, 103

Genetic causes, 2, 11

Glucagon, 16, 60, 99, 119

Glycogen, 70

Growth, 52

"Growth spurts," 30

Healthy body weight, 37

    attaining, 46, 67, 88-89

Healthy eating. *See* Eating healthy foods

Home schooling, 34

Hunger, 52

Hyperglycemia, 25, 80, 98

    recognizing an emergency, 120

Hyperinsulinemia, 97

Hypoglycemia, 5-6, 8, 25, 40, 79, 98

    preventing, 26, 45, 65, 70

    signs of low blood glucose, 119

    treating, 14, 16, 60

    unawareness of, 74, 82, 98

Infants with diabetes, 13-19

    small insulin adjustments for, 17

Insulin pens, 56, 59

Insulin pumps, 17, 56-57, 70

    for toddlers, 63

    for young athletes, 104

Insulin resistance, 30, 37

    acanthosis nigricans in, 97

    PCOS in, 41

    puberty in, 39

Insulin therapy, 2

    adjusting, 71

    administering, 56

    "honeymoon" phase, 62

    lowering for active periods, 6, 70-71, 103-104

    oral, 61

    skipping doses of, 36, 89

    types of, 17, 55, 57-58

Jet injectors, 56

Ketones, 69

    testing for, 80

Lifestyle changes, 3-4, 97

Log book records, 81

Marijuana use, 123

Mealtimes, 19

    handling refusal to eat, 22

Medical alert identification, 6, 25, 106, 112, 121

Medications, 4, 25

    managing, 55-64

    oral, 61

Menstrual periods, and diabetes, 40

Mental health professionals. *See* Counseling assistance

Metformin, 61

Microalbuminuria, 64

Monitoring. *See* Blood glucose monitoring

Nap time, 15

Nephropathy, 36, 64

Neuropathy, 36

Non-nutritive sweeteners, 50

Nutrient requirements, 51

Nutrition Facts labels, 48

Obesity, 2, 5, 11. *See also* Healthy body weight

Pacific Islander youth, with diabetes, 11
Pancreas transplants, 4
Parents
    feeling overwhelmed, 10
    "job description," 22
    remaining flexible, 27, 32
    sharing responsibility for diabetes care,
        33, 106, 116
Parties, suggestions for, 49
Peer pressure, 107
"Percentile for weight" measurements, 36
Physical activity and exercise, 25, 65-72, 99
    increasing, 3-4, 37
    lack of, 2, 11
    suggestions for, 66-67
Pizza, effect on blood glucose levels, 111
Play therapy, 7
Polycystic ovarian syndrome (PCOS), 41
Portion sizes, 46-49
"Positive reinforcement," 23
Praising children, 8, 19, 23
Pregnancy, and diabetes, 38
Psychological help. See Counseling assistance
Puberty, effect on insulin resistance, 39

Racial aspects. See individual racial and
        ethnic groups
"Rebounding," 82
Rehabilitation Act of 1973, 94
Restaurant dining, suggestions for, 49
Retinopathy, 36
Rewarding children, 7
    using non-food items, 23

Safety issues, 25, 105
    recognizing an emergency, 120
    risky behaviors by youngsters, 123
    on the school bus, 96
    signs of low blood glucose, 119
School-aged children with diabetes, 29-34
School and school activities, 31, 34, 86,
        93-99. See also Athletes with diabetes
    sick days, 118

Self-esteem, 107
    strengthening, 29, 88
Self-identity, 107
    developing, 35
Self-management. See Diabetes self-management
Self-monitoring of blood glucose (SBMG),
        73-74, 77, 83
Smoking, 123
Snacks, 6, 45
    setting out clear guidelines for, 26
    skipping, 26
    suggestions for, 45
Social difficulties, risk for, 31, 53, 85-91
Social situations, 107-113
Softball, and diabetes, 104
Sports drinks, 72
Sugar, 44, 46
    children craving, 32
    not causing diabetes, 1-11
"Sugar-free" foods and beverages, 50, 72
Support groups, 10, 88
Sweeteners, non-nutritive, 50

Toddlers with diabetes, 13-19, 58
    caregivers for, 18
    handling power struggles, 19, 21
Trauma of injections and finger sticks, 7, 79
    minimizing, 15
Traveling, preparing for, 112
Trick-or-treating, 113
Type 1 diabetes, vii, 11, 74, 89
Type 2 diabetes, vii, 11, 75
    treating in children, vii, 30, 66, 88

Unpredictability, 27

Vitamins and minerals, 50

Worry, preventing needless, 38

Young children with diabetes, 21-27

About the American Diabetes Association

The American Diabetes Association is the nation's leading voluntary health organization supporting diabetes research, information, and advocacy. Its mission is to prevent and cure diabetes and to improve the lives of all people affected by diabetes. The American Diabetes Association is the leading publisher of comprehensive diabetes information. Its huge library of practical and authoritative books for people with diabetes covers every aspect of self-care—cooking and nutrition, fitness, weight control, medications, complications, emotional issues, and general self-care.

To order American Diabetes Association books: Call 1-800-232-6733 or log on to http://store.diabetes.org

To join the American Diabetes Association: Call 1-800-806-7801 or log on to www.diabetes.org/membership

For more information about diabetes or ADA programs and services: Call 1-800-342-2383. E-mail: AskADA@diabetes.org or log on to www.diabetes.org

To locate an ADA/NCQA Recognized Provider of quality diabetes care in your area: www.ncqa.org/dprp

To find an ADA Recognized Education Program in your area: Call 1-800-342-2383. www.diabetes.org/for-health-professionals-and-scientists/recognition/edrecognition.jsp

To join the fight to increase funding for diabetes research, end discrimination, and improve insurance coverage: Call 1-800-342-2383. www.diabetes.org/advocacy-and-legalresources/advocacy.jsp

To find out how you can get involved with the programs in your community: Call 1-800-342-2383. See below for program Web addresses.

American Diabetes Month: educational activities aimed at those diagnosed with diabetes—month of November. www.diabetes.org/communityprograms-and-localevents/americandiabetesmonth.jsp

American Diabetes Alert: annual public awareness campaign to find the undiagnosed—held the fourth Tuesday in March. www.diabetes.org/communityprograms-and-localevents/americandiabetesalert.jsp

The Diabetes Assistance & Resources Program (DAR): diabetes awareness program targeted to the Latino community. www.diabetes.org/communityprograms-and-localevents/latinos.jsp

African American Program: diabetes awareness program targeted to the African American community. www.diabetes.org/communityprograms-and-localevents/africanamericans.jsp

Awakening the Spirit: Pathways to Diabetes Prevention & Control: diabetes awareness program targeted to the Native American community. www.diabetes.org/communityprograms-and-localevents/nativeamericans.jsp

To find out about an important research project regarding type 2 diabetes: www.diabetes.org/diabetes-research/research-home.jsp

To obtain information on making a planned gift or charitable bequest: Call 1-888-700-7029. www.wpg.cc/stl/CDA/homepage/1,1006,509,00.html

To make a donation or memorial contribution: Call 1-800-342-2383. www.diabetes.org/support-the-cause/make-a-donation.jsp